the
master
cleanse
made easy

the
master
cleanse
made easy

Your No-Fail Guide to Feeling Great During and After the Detox

Robin Westen

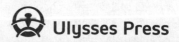 Ulysses Press

Published in the US by
ULYSSES PRESS
P.O. Box 3440
Berkeley, CA 94703
www.ulyssespress.com

ISBN: 978-1-61243-400-1
Library of Congress Control Number 2014943032

10 9 8 7 6 5 4 3 2 1

Printed in Canada by Marquis Book Printing

Acquisitions Editor: Katherine Furman
Managing Editor: Claire Chun
Editor: Renee Rutledge
Proofreader: Lauren Harrison
Layout: Lindsay Tamura
Indexer: Sayre Van Young
Front Cover Design: Rebecca Lown
Front Cover Photo: lemon © azure1/shutterstock.com

Distributed by Publishers Group West

NOTE TO READERS: This book has been written and published
strictly for informational and educational purposes only. It is not
intended to serve as medical advice or to be any form of medical
treatment. You should always consult your physician before altering
or changing any aspect of your medical treatment and/or undertaking
a diet regimen, including the guidelines as described in this book. Do
not stop or change any prescription medications without the guidance
and advice of your physician. Any use of the information in this book
is made on the reader's good judgment after consulting with his
or her physician and is the reader's sole responsibility. This book is
not intended to diagnose or treat any medical condition and is not a
substitute for a physician.

For Dr. Bebop, always

table of contents

introduction

I went on my first detox cleanse more than a decade ago. In those days, I was a real beginner. Not knowing much about what I was getting myself into, but aware that I really needed to do something about the state of my body and mind, I chose the Master Cleanse (MC), also known as the Lemonade Diet. For over 70 years, thousands of people from all over the world have been doing the same.

There are plenty of reasons for choosing the MC; it's simple, inexpensive, and awesomely effective. It improves health by drastically detoxing your system, and as a result boosts your physical and emotional well-being. The truth is, although the Master Cleanse was remarkably beneficial for me and one of the initial influences in my quest to live a balanced and abundant life, it also presented intense challenges and had a few drawbacks. That's why I decided to write this book. If you choose to go on the Master Cleanse, this will prepare you fully, with awareness of the challenges, strategies to stay the course, and techniques to ease out with grace once the 10 days come to a close.

From the beginning, the MC was controversial. Its creator, Stanley Burroughs (also known as Aaron Hayes), faced skepticism when he introduced the cleanse in the 1940s. Already a controversial figure for championing unconventional approaches to different modalities and healing techniques, Burroughs was an advocate of color therapy, deep massage, and reflexology, a practice that was little known in the West at the time. He was also a strict vegetarian and a devout nudist. More damaging was the fact that Burroughs proclaimed himself a healer. His legal downfall came when he used his lemonade detox cleanse, or Lemonade Diet, on a patient dying of cancer. This landed him in front of the California Supreme Court on second-degree felony murder charges. He was convicted of practicing medicine without a license and spent several years in prison. In 1991, Burroughs died at the age of 88.

Well, that's a brief look at Burroughs's complicated life. But this book is all about *your* life and how your journey with the Master Cleanse can be so much easier and safer. You'll gain:

- tips on how to ease in and out of the cleanse;
- step-by-step instructions on creating the MC lemonade (as well as the saltwater flush, which pushes toxins from your system) and following the cleanse regimen;
- information about the trials *you* may face while trying to stick to the cleanse;
- specific solutions to help you through those tough spots;

- descriptions of numerous complementary therapies; and
- follow-up recipes to stay detoxed while maintaining weight loss.

When instructions of the cleanse are not followed, potential dangers include: developing a dependence on laxatives; electrolyte imbalance; dehydration; and the rare chance of developing metabolic acidosis, a high level of acid in your blood. But these conditions are nearly always the result of not following the Master Cleanse as directed, or staying on it too long.

Several quizzes are included to give you insight into your personal strengths and weaknesses. While priming to follow through on the MC's rigorous program, it's crucial to be aware of the toxic forces at play in your daily life. Chapter One describes our toxic world and why a fresh start with the Master Cleanse is so critical. The quiz, "What's Your Toxicity Level?" on page 30, will indicate the most toxic areas of your life, providing instant cleansing strategies to complement the MC.

In Chapter Two, you'll discover how and why the MC works and get an overview of the short- and long-term benefits you can expect. Find out why ingredients of the MC (water, lemons, pepper, and maple syrup) are so powerful, and learn what to expect physically, mentally, and emotionally while you're on the cleanse. Take the quiz, "How Ready Are You for the Master Cleanse?" on page 48. Your score will reveal those aspects of the MC that will benefit you most, as well as your vulnerability to possible complications, followed by advice on how to avoid them. If you're interested in the

Hollywood crowd, I'll give you the scoop on which stars have benefited from Burroughs's program.

Simple instructions on how to prepare for the MC, including what to cut out the week prior, how to read instructions, what you'll need to buy, and suggested activities (including avoiding exercise and taking a sauna) are described in Chapter Three. Plus, you'll learn "selfie" techniques you can do in your own home, from body scrubs to lymphatic massage, and simple Do's and Don'ts. The quiz, "Test Your MC Know-How" on page 63, will clue you in on how much information about the cleanse you've retained so far and give you a chance to brush up on information you might have missed.

Chapter Four gives you everything you need to know about making the MC lemonade concoction, your primary source of nutrition during the MC, and the saltwater flush (SWF). Learn the importance of taking a daily natural laxative while you're on the MC, and get tips on how to stay on track, including ways to boost your motivation, resist temptation, and cut cravings. The quiz, "Discover Your Strongest Suit and Overcome Obstacles" on page 81, identifies a personal "gift" that will enable you to stick to the MC, even at its most challenging. Complementary techniques focusing on emotions such as forgiveness and gratitude are also found here.

Let me remind you here, knowledge really is power. Chapter Five provides a day-by-day look at what you'll be going through, along with insight on the importance of sticking to the cleanse for 10 full days. I also describe the most common side effects—both pleasant and unpleasant—of the cleanse. Tips in this chapter highlight other ways to detox, including tongue scraping, opening your heart chakra, and Metta meditation. Take the quiz, "What's Your Innate Ability to Meet Challenges?" on page 101, and tune in to your strongest personality traits.

Chapter Six will be crucial in helping you ease out of the cleanse gently after your 10 days are up. By this time, you'll feel super good and might be tempted to stay longer on the cleanse. Yes, believe it or not, it happens. But you're encouraged to end it now and end it slowly. A recipe for a light, delicious vegetable soup is offered to prepare your tummy for more strenuous digestion in the days to come. You'll also get a look at superfoods and how they affect your body. Plus, you'll be given a heads-up on some foods you should seriously avoid. There are also plenty of suggestions for activities that will enhance the end of your cleanse. Your score on the quiz, "Are You Nice Enough to Yourself?" on page 120, lets you know if more TLC is called for, with suggestions on how to make that happen.

Chapter Seven's recipes for breakfast, lunch, and dinner, as well as a variety of healthy snacks, will help you maintain a state of detox and hold on to most of your weight loss. Tips on what to do when you're dining out and other strategies for healthy eating can be found here, along with a special section on boosting mood.

The last chapter offers methods outside dietary cleansing to take care of your body, mind, and spirit, including aromatherapy, bathing, a restorative yoga pose, and ways to remain mindful. You'll find the quiz "Calculate Your Energy Quotient" on page 172, with subsequent tips on how to keep buzzing.

Even with careful preparation, helpful tips, Do's and Don'ts, revealing quizzes, and the easy and yummy recipes offered in the upcoming pages, you still might find the Master Cleanse too tough a detox program to follow. Don't be hard on yourself. Give yourself another chance. Open up to change, envision yourself detoxed and healthy—and then see what happens. If you still want out, that's okay, too. There are other options available. Consider reading my other books, *The 2-Day Superfood Cleanse* or *The Yoga-Body Cleanse.* Both of the programs are shorter and easier to maintain because they're not fasts but detox diets that include eating foods.

Ultimately, the most important lesson to be learned from your detox journey is the ability to tune in to yourself. Your mind, body, and spirit are there to help. Listen up—and enjoy life.

one

do *you* need the master cleanse?

> We need to accept the seemingly obvious fact that a toxic environment can make people sick and that no amount of medical intervention can protect us.
>
> —ANDREW WEIL, MD AND NATUROPATH

We live in a dirty world. Our air, water, and food (even some so-called organic foods) can be minefields of poison. Add stress to the mix, as well as other unhealthy emotions and lifestyle habits, and *whoa*—you're frolicking in a toxic playground.

Exactly What Is a Toxin?

According to *Merriam-Webster's Collegiate Dictionary*, a toxin is "a poisonous substance that is a specific product of the metabolic activities of a living organism and is usually very unstable, notably toxic when introduced into the tissues, and typically capable of inducing antibody formation." Or to put it another way, toxins attack our physical, spiritual, mental, and emotional being. Everything.

Toxins can make you feel sick and look awful, dampen your enthusiasm, and suck your energy. Toxins may be responsible for headaches, fatigue, mood disorders, tummy aches, fuzzy thinking, aching muscles, a compromised immune system, and inflammation in the body (which can lead to tissue damage, heart disease, and arthritis, just to name a few complications).

The good news? *Yes*, good news. Toxicity doesn't have to take over your life. You can get rid of it. You can clear out the toxins, repair the damage, renew your spirit, spark your energy, and gain back your youthful appearance, all the while losing extra thigh-thickening pounds. The answer is the Master Cleanse, the absolute gold standard of cleanses. It's been around for decades and its amazing benefits are world-renowned.

• •

Can Anyone Go on the Master Cleanse?

No! Folks with diabetes, cancer, anemia, intestinal obstruction, or gallstones, or those who are underweight, have an eating disorder, or are pregnant or nursing should definitely *not* go on the Master Cleanse. If you have *any* doubts, or are on medication(s), speak with your doctor about going on the MC.

• •

Toxic Enemies

Before we get into the nitty-gritty of this amazing cleansing program, it's a good idea to identify the major toxic forces contributing to what may be your less-than-optimal health.

What You Eat

Salmonella. Salmonella is usually found in poultry, eggs, unprocessed milk, meat, and water. Each year, according to the Centers for Disease Control and Prevention (CDC), it's estimated that salmonella causes about 1.2 million illnesses in the United States, with about 23,000 hospitalizations and 450 deaths. Most folks infected with salmonella develop diarrhea, fever, and abdominal cramps 12 to 72 hours after infection. The salmonella infection can spread from the intestines to the bloodstream, and then to other body sites, and can even cause death unless the person is treated promptly with antibiotics. The elderly, infants, and people with impaired immune systems are more likely to suffer the most.

E. coli (Escherichia coli). This is bacteria that under the right circumstances live happily in our intestines. And most kinds of E. coli won't hurt you. That said, some strains can lead to serious anemia, kidney failure, or even death. You can get this toxic infection if you come into contact with the feces (stool) of humans or animals; it can happen when you drink liquids or eat food that has been contaminated. Most commonly, the contamination happens during meat processing, but it can also happen in agricultural fields and when food is prepared in restaurants. Besides meat, other common culprits include dairy products (especially raw milk), fruits and vegetables such as lettuce or alfalfa sprouts, or unpasteurized juices that have come in contact with infected feces.

FYI: Think before you swim. E. coli sometimes get into lakes, ponds, and pools.

Parasites. These are organisms that can live in our intestines and consume nutrients. They usually invade our system through food and water, often while we're traveling in foreign countries with less-than-satisfactory sanitation systems. But you can also pick up parasites when you're eating out at your favorite restaurants.

Pesticides. Shockingly, the Environmental Protection Agency (EPA) warns us that 60 percent of herbicides, 90 percent of fungicides, and 30 percent of insecticides are known to be carcinogenic—and yet, they're still prevalent in our food supplies. In fact, pesticide residues have been detected in 50 to 95 percent of our foods. They're in our fruits, veggies, and meats and can put us at risk for miscarriage, nerve damage, birth defects, and a gut that can't absorb the nutrients in food.

Hormones. Most of the commercial livestock in our country have synthetic hormones in their feed, and the most common one is estrogen. Women need this hormone for their reproductive systems, as well as to control bone growth and cholesterol levels. But as reported by the *Oxford Journals*, too much estrogen has been linked to breast, prostate, and endometrial cancers. Hormones increase the chances of cancer, thyroid disease, diabetes, obesity, infertility, asthma, and allergies.

Heavy metals. Arsenic is routinely added to chicken feed by the food industry. All farmed fish or even wild fish (excluding wild sockeye salmon) have high levels of mercury and toxins in them.

Genetically modified foods (GMOs). Even though genetically modified foods have been approved by the government and certified to be safe, there are several types of potential health effects that could result from putting a novel gene into an organism. This is especially evident in our food supply. So far there's been evidence, as reported by the Institute for Responsible Technology, the University of Minnesota School of Public Health, and *Oxford Journals*, to name a few, that GMO foods are responsible for the production of new allergens (peanut allergies, anyone?), increased toxicity, decreased nutrition, and antibiotic resistance.

••

Since 1996, bacteria, viruses, and other genes have been artificially inserted to the DNA of soy, corn, cottonseed, and canola plants.

••

PCBs (polychlorinated biphenyls). This industrial chemical has been banned in the United States for decades, yet it continues to be an organic pollutant that's prevalent in our environment. It's most commonly found in farm-raised salmon. According to GreenFacts.org, 50 studies conducted since 1976 have pointed to the role of PCBs in cancer, impaired fetal brain development, and other serious health concerns.

Phthalates. These chemicals are used to soften plastics and are hugely responsible for the downside of bottled water. Phthalates can do damage to our endocrine system because they chemically mimic hormones and may be particularly dangerous to children. In addition to plastic bottles, this toxin is found most commonly in plastic wraps and plastic food-storage containers, all of which leach phthalates into our food.

Butylated hydroxytoluene, butylated hydroxyanisole, and tertiary butylhydroquinone (BHT, BHA, and TBHQ). These chemicals are used to help keep fats in foods from going rancid. They've been linked with serious concerns like increasing cancer risk, disrupting estrogen balance, asthma, and hyperactivity. They're often added to cereal, nut mixes, gum, butter, meat, and dehydrated potatoes.

Perfluorooctanoic acid (PFOA). The paper and lining of microwave popcorn bags contain PFOAs. At high heats, like those created in your microwave, PFOAs vaporize and spread into the food, most frequently with popcorn. PFOAs can also be inhaled through the steam given off if the bag of microwave popcorn is opened too quickly after heating. PFOA has been linked by the American Cancer Society to thyroid disease in humans and cancers in animals.

Azodicarbonamide. This is a bleaching agent used in packaged and processed foods like frozen dinners and pasta, as well as flour mixes in baked goods. Various studies, including those conducted by the World Health Organization, link the toxic chemical to cancer risk and asthma.

Chloroform. This toxic ingredient is mostly formed when chlorine is added to water. It's in our air and drinking water, as well as in our food supply. It can put people at risk for potential reproductive damage, birth defects, dizziness, fatigue, headache, liver and kidney damage, and cancer. It's also found in our water supply and escapes into the air.

Bisphenol (BPA). This is an estrogen-like chemical that's pervasive in canned foods. BPA is linked to a wide array of health concerns including reproductive problems; cancer risk; metabolic disorders such as obesity, type 2 diabetes, and insulin resistance; heart disease; and neurobehavioral effects, most commonly ADHD. BPA is particularly risky in canned tomatoes because the acidity of the tomato can leach even more of this toxin into the food.

Food dyes. Even though the European Union put regulations on labeling food dyes so their consumers will know what they're eating, this is not so in the United States. These are the most common food dyes used in our food supply today:

- *Blue #1.* A Center for Science in the Public Interest study point to Blue #1 causing kidney tumors in mice. It's found in baked goods, beverages, dessert powders, candies, cereal, medications, and other products.
- *Blue #2.* This has been shown to cause tumors, particularly brain gliomas in male rats. It's found in colored beverages, candies and other foods, pet food, and medications.
- *Citrus Red #2.* This has been found to cause tumors in the bladder of rats. Shockingly, Citrus Red #2 is in the skins of Florida oranges.
- *Green #3.* This has caused significant increases in bladder and testes tumors in male rats. It's found

in beverages, ice cream, and sorbet, as well as in lipsticks and plenty of externally applied cosmetics.

- *Red #3 (Erythrosine).* Recognized in 1990 by the FDA as a thyroid carcinogen in animals and now banned in cosmetics, this is still in sausage casings, maraschino cherries, baked goods, and candies.

- *Red #40 (Allura Red).* This is the most widely used and consumed dye. It may accelerate the appearance of immune system tumors in mice. It causes hypersensitivity (allergy-like) reactions in some consumers and might trigger hyperactivity in children. Studies by the Center for Science in the Public Interest show it could be responsible for contributing to immune system tumors in mice. It's found in beverages, baked goods, dessert powders, candies, and cereals.

- *Yellow #5.* This dye can cause sometimes severe hypersensitivity reactions and might trigger hyperactivity and other behavioral effects in children. It's found in numerous baked goods, beverages, dessert powders, candies, cereals, gelatin desserts, and many other foods.

- *Yellow #6.* This has caused adrenal tumors in animals and occasionally causes severe hypersensitivity reactions. It's found in baked goods, cereals, beverages, dessert powders, candies, gelatin deserts, and sausage, as well as cosmetics and medications.

FYI: US manufacturers drench 15 million pounds of artificial food dyes into our diets every year.

What You Breathe

Mold and other fungal toxins. These can be found in contaminated buildings, foods like peanuts, wheat, and corn, and in alcoholic beverages. Mycotoxins (fungal toxins) may cause a range of health problems, from cancer and heart disease to asthma, multiple sclerosis, and diabetes. Exposure to even a small amount can damage your health. In fact, statistics show one in three people have had an allergic reaction to mold.

Volatile organic compounds (VOCs). These are big contributing factors to the destruction of our ozone layer. According to the EPA, VOCs tend to be even higher (two to five times) in indoor air than outdoor air because they're present in so many household cleaning products. VOCs have been linked by the US National Library of Medicine to cancer, eye, and respiratory tract irritation, headaches, dizziness, visual disorders, and memory impairment. They're found in carpeting, paints, deodorants, cleaning fluids, varnishes, cosmetics, dry-cleaned clothing, moth repellents, air fresheners, and even in our drinking water.

Asbestos. Most of us know by now how dangerous asbestos is, but that doesn't help to solve the problem. Used primarily as an insulating material between the 1950s and the 1970s (before it was banned), asbestos is still found in insulation on floors, ceilings, water pipes, and heating ducts that were built during that period. When these materials start to decompose, the fibers release into the air and can put people at risk for lung tissue scarring and mesothelioma (a rare form of cancer).

Dioxins. These are chemical compounds created by combustion processes such as commercial or municipal waste incineration, as well as from burning fuels like wood, oil, or coal. Dioxins have been linked by the EPA and the US National Toxicology Program to cancer, reproductive, and developmental disorders, skin rashes, skin discoloration, excessive body hair, and mild liver damage.

Chlorine. Despite the fact that chlorine is a highly toxic gas that can cause sore throat, coughing, eye and skin irritation, rapid breathing, narrowing of the bronchi, wheezing, blue coloring of the skin, accumulation of fluid in the lungs, pain in the lung region, severe eye and skin burns, lung collapse, and a type of asthma called reactive airways dysfunction syndrome (RADS), it's widely used. It can be found in household cleaners and in the air (when near certain industries such as paper plants), as well as in limited amounts in drinking water.

What You Feel

Stress and anxiety. In the old days we really needed stress to survive. That's because major stress triggers our body's response, known as the fight-or-flight response, to a perceived threat or danger. This was helpful when we had to be vigilant to survive, but in our modern lives this kind of hyper stress reaction does more harm than good. During the fight-or-flight response certain hormones like adrenalin and cortisol are released, speeding our heart rate, slowing digestion, shunting blood flow to major muscle groups, and changing various other autonomic nervous functions, as well as giving us a burst of energy and strength we don't really need. When stress is ongoing in our lives we end up with an over-activated autonomic nervous system. It's a toxic reaction.

Hopelessness and depression. For many Americans, chronic unhappiness can seem to be a normal state. The effects of hopelessness and depression create a toxic environment that exists not only in our minds, but also in our bodies. The symptoms of its toxicity include gaining or losing weight, sleeplessness or sleeping too much, eating lots of junk food or loss of appetite, not having the energy to exercise, isolation from friends and loved ones, or, at its worst, losing interest in life itself. The good news is that the Master Cleanse boosts moods by clearing out blockages in organs and allowing the smooth flow of life-affirming energy.

Anger. When was the last time you were angry—really fuming? Did you let it out in a gust of fury, or did you keep it to yourself, silently smoldering? Either way, anger is toxic. Your body responded with a surge in hormones, your heart rate went on a gallop, and your breathing got faster. What's more, there's a good chance your blood pressure shot up (because your blood vessels restrict), though, hopefully not to a boiling point. That's because similar to the stress reaction, when you're angry your fight-or-flight response is triggered. In fact, researchers believe that frequent anger may speed up the process of atherosclerosis, a condition that leads to hardening and blockage of the arteries. BTW: High levels of anxiety and depression have also been found to contribute to an increased risk for heart disease.

Fives Questions That Can Help Calm Anger

- What is this going to mean to me two months from now—even tomorrow?
- What am I accomplishing by being angry?
- Is there another way I can deal with this problem?
- How do I want others to perceive me?
- What do I gain if I blame someone else for what I'm feeling?

The Master Cleanse will flush out any lingering anger and wipe your "emotional slate" clean. But realistically, this feeling of unconditional bliss may only linger for a week or two beyond the Master Cleanse. If you think you may suffer from a more serious anger problem, you may want to consider counseling or anger management. Speak with your medical advisor about finding the counseling option that is right for you.

Jealousy and envy. Strictly speaking, jealousy and envy are defined differently, but ultimately, they cause the same kinds of destructive shock waves to your body. Psychologists describe envy as directed at another or others—wanting their qualities, success, or possession. Jealousy, on the other hand, involves thinking you will lose, or have lost, some affection or security from another person because of someone or something else, including their interest in an activity that takes time away from you. But both jealousy and envy share common ground because each involves comparisons and contrasts.

Whatever the trigger, just as the other emotions described above, envy and jealousy are forms of energy that run through your body like an electrical current. As the electrical current of an emotion travels along your neural pathways, it triggers the release of chemical proteins called neuropeptides (NPs). Adrenalin, hormones, oxytocin, endorphins—these are all NPs. Each neuropeptide creates such specific biological responses that physical symptoms such as indigestion (in the case of jealousy or envy) and heart disease (in the case of anger) can actually point to what's really going on in your unconscious mind.

The Benefit of Bliss

Happiness, joy, and laughter, as well as orgasms, cause the release of endorphins. Endorphins are powerful opiates that make you feel good. They boost your immune system, relax muscles, elevate your mood, and dampen pain.

Your Body's Super-Cleansing Systems

You'll probably be happy to learn your body isn't just hanging out passively waiting for the "Attack of the Toxins." It's built with natural purifying systems. When they're overwhelmed, it's time for the Master Cleanse!

Kidneys. Your two kidneys work to purify your blood and remove excess water, salts, bile pigments, and cellular wastes for excretion (through your urine). This process is the reason why getting enough water is so important. Water is the transportation system that carries toxins to your kidneys and helps to flush them out. The more water you drink, the more you'll excrete toxins from your body.

FYI: For optimum health, drink at least six 8-ounce glasses of water every day. More when you're cleansing, exercising, or on hot days when you sweat more.

Liver. There's an expression "Love your liver, live longer," and for good reason. The rock star of your body's detox system is the liver. That's because the liver produces good bile to break down bad fats. It also helps to detoxify drugs, alcohol, and other particularly harsh toxins. But if you abuse your liver by overloading it with the bad stuff, it will eventually just give up. That's why it's so important to give your liver a break every now and then by engaging in the Master Cleanse. While you're on the cleanse, your liver can just relax and rejuvenate.

Skin. Your skin is your largest organ and it works as a detox system, removing urea (protein metabolism), as well as salts and water. How does it do it? Through sweat. That's why exercising and saunas are so good for you.

Colon. Your colon (or large intestine) acts like a slide for stool to exit your body. Through elimination of fecal matter, wastes are removed from your body on a daily basis. If there is slow movement, stool can back up and sit longer in your colon than it was intended. This can lead to the discomfort associated with gas, cramping, and bloating. It can also allow those waste products, such as estrogens and other metabolites, to be reabsorbed into the body. Sluggish colonic activity can predispose people to colon cancer, especially if there's family history of the illness.

FYI: Beware of antibiotics! Yes, when you really need them, they can save your life—and in those cases don't hesitate to take them. But understand that in the process of killing bad bacteria, antibiotics also kill the good stuff, specifically the flora in our guts that we need to be healthy. This can contribute to everything from yeast infection to depression. The rule: Don't take antibiotics indiscriminately and avoid soaps and other products with antibacterial ingredients.

Quiz: What's Your Toxicity Level?

You might be wondering just where you stand on the toxicity scale. After all, not everyone's lifestyle is the same; some of us are more susceptible to certain temptations, while others may have weaker immune systems. Before moving on to the next chapter, where you'll read about the ins and outs of the Master Cleanse, take this quiz to discover your starting point. Based on your score, you'll also get some quick cleansing tips. You might want to try them before beginning your Master Cleanse.

	Frequently	Rarely	Never
Do you have headaches?	O	O	O
Do you suffer with allergies?	O	O	O
Do you have dark circles under your eyes?	O	O	O
Do you crave sugary foods?	O	O	O
Do you have a hard time sleeping?	O	O	O
Or do you sleep too much?	O	O	O
Do you have pain or stiffness in your joints?	O	O	O
Do you get bloated after eating?	O	O	O
Do you have difficult bowel movements?	O	O	O
Or do you suffer with bouts of diarrhea?	O	O	O

Do you catch colds?	○	○	○
Do you have fuzzy brain?	○	○	○
Do you suffer with bouts of depression or anxiety?	○	○	○
Do you take over-the-counter or prescription medications?	○	○	○
Do you use toxic cleaning supplies?	○	○	○
Are you sensitive to scents?	○	○	○
Do you get enraged?	○	○	○
Do you have trouble with your memory?	○	○	○
Do you overeat?	○	○	○
Do you get heartburn?	○	○	○

Scoring

Give yourself 5 points for every *Frequently* answer, 3 points for *Rarely*, and 0 points for *Never*. Add your points.

Between 75 and 100 points: High on the Toxicity Scale

Your score shows that your symptoms, as well as your lifestyle, point to an overload of toxicity. On the upside, this also means that you'll benefit the most from the Master Cleanse, which has been shown to remedy many of these conditions. But in order for it to be successful you'll need to make a commitment to change many of the choices you're making in your daily life—before and after the Master Cleanse. This may include reducing or eliminating alcohol, sugar, caffeine, and processed foods, as well as nixing any toxic cleaning products. You'll also benefit from:

- Daily walks in the sunshine, which will boost your mood and positive outlook, and help you sleep through the night so you'll have energy for the cleanse.
- Keeping a food journal, which can help identify those foods that may be causing you particular discomfort. As soon as they're identified, eliminate them for good.
- Encouraging a friend to join you in the Master Cleanse, which can help to keep your motivation strong. Studies show dieting with a friend increases chances of sticking with it.

Between 30 and 74 points: Midway on the Toxicity Scale

Depending on where you scored within this range of points, you're dealing with a certain level of toxicity that may, or may not, be apparent to you. The issues you may be dealing with can include frequent colds, puffy eyes, or food cravings, symptoms you might just take for granted because they're life as you know it. Well, that needn't be the case. The Master Cleanse can change your life. Before you begin, you might want to:

- Take a sauna to sweat out deep toxins.
- Engage in 15 minutes of mindfulness meditation to open your awareness of the present so you can notice the changes.
- Try tai chi or yoga as a way to keep your body flexible and receptive.

Fewer Than 29 points: Low on the Toxicity Scale

Everyone has *some* toxicity. But considering all the negative dietary and environmental influences in our modern lives, if this is your score range, you're doing pretty well. Chances are you've been paying attention to what your physical, mental, emotional, and spiritual needs are. Good for you! Still, everyone can benefit from doing the Master Cleanse at least once or twice a year. You may discover yourself entering a whole new realm of health you didn't even know existed. For now:

- Engage in deep breathing. Your body is designed to release 70 percent of its toxins through breathing. When you exhale air from your body, you release carbon dioxide that has been passed from your bloodstream into your lungs. Carbon dioxide is a natural waste of your body's metabolism.
- Stretch. It increases circulation and can bump up your detox.
- Give yourself a pat on the back for taking such good care of yourself. You deserve it.

•••••••••••

two

the master of all cleanses

Krishna insisted on outer cleanliness and inner cleansing. Clean clothes and clean minds are an ideal combination.

—SRI SATHYA SAI BABA
(INDIAN SPIRITUAL LEADER)

The Ins and Outs of the MC

There's no secret to the MC. It's simple, direct, and pure, and its healing results, both internal and external, are undeniable. In very basic terms the Master Cleanse, which has been around for over 70 years, can be considered a modified 10-day juice cleanse. That's because you'll be drinking a healing potion of lemonade made with lemon, maple syrup, cayenne pepper, and water. You'll find the exact recipe for the concoction in Chapter Four, but right now, just know that it involves drinking six to twelve glasses of the liquid (which includes water, the juice of three to six lemons, and one-half to three-fourths of a cup of maple syrup).

The Master Cleanse does *not* require:

- A big expense—ingredients are few and inexpensive
- Major preparation—it's a snap to create
- Physical exertion—just relax, breathe, and meditate

Plus, it's good for vegans and vegetarians and it's kosher, halal, and gluten-free!

Note: As part of the daily routine, an herbal laxative and saltwater drink are also recommended.

How the MC Can Change Your Life

The Master Cleanse benefits include detoxing your organs big time as well as removing excess fat from your body. These effects will make you look, feel, and *be* healthier. They will lead to a dramatic increase in your energy levels, enable you to get rid of unhealthy lifestyle habits, boost your metabolism rate, cleanse your kidneys and digestive system, purify the glands and cells throughout your body, eliminate unusable waste and hardened material in your joints and muscles, build a healthier bloodstream, and bring back a youthful elasticity and glow to your skin.

How great is that?

The caveat: You need to be ready and open to make changes in your life in order for the MC to work its wonders; you need to be willing to go through the detox-ification process, which may not always be so pleasant. Downside: You'll have to do without eating meals for 10 days.

Upside: Surprisingly, for most of the detox period, you won't be hungry. You'll feel super-energetic, and after a few days, you'll look like you just stepped out of a spa.

Benefits of the Master Cleanse include:

- Improved bowel function
- Clearer skin
- Better mental clarity and concentration
- Fewer headaches
- Less bloating
- Reduced indigestion and acid reflux
- Better ability to absorb nutrients
- A sense of well-being and calm
- Improvement of conditions like allergies and asthma
- Higher energy levels
- Lower blood pressure

Big-Time Weight Loss

The MC's daily caloric intake is only between 650 and 1,300 calories, depending on how many glasses of the lemonade you choose to drink. Most folks who haven't packed on too many extra pounds need between 1,600 to 2,400 calories daily to keep their weight stable. So there's a pretty good chance you'll lose at least five to eight pounds of fat during the 10-day program and considerably more in water weight. With this in mind, some cleansers report losing 20 pounds in 10 days—and that's not surprising. But realistically, you'll probably gain most of the water weight back pretty soon after the cleanse is over.

Star Power

The Master Cleanse not only has fans—but star power, too! Check out these mega-celebs who also did the detox. Master Cleanse Celebrities:

- Beyoncé Knowles (who dropped 20 pounds in two weeks for her role in the movie *Dreamgirls*
- Robin Quivers, Howard Stern's sidekick
- Gwyneth Paltrow
- Ashanti
- Jared Leto
- David Blaine
- Demi Moore
- Naomi Campbell
- Eddie Vedder
- Josh Brolin
- Ashton Kutcher
- Heidi Klum

Protein Power

Even though the MC offers several hundred calories of carbs every day thanks to its fresh lemon and maple syrup, there's obviously no meat, dairy, tofu, or beans. Burroughs informed followers not to be concerned since protein is simply a combination of oxygen, hydrogen, carbon, and nitrogen. And guess what contains all these elements? The air you breathe! He once said that just by breathing in and out, "we are able to assimilate and build the nitrogen in our bodies as protein." Science may disagree. I'm just putting it out there.

Vitamin C Sensation!

The Master Cleanse is also super high in vitamin C. That's why while you're on the MC you'll gain brighter and clearer skin, healthier gums, and a stronger immune system.

Scientific Studies: Eat a Lot Less, Live a Lot Longer

Research is leaning toward the conclusion that the less we consume, the longer we'll be around to enjoy life. You might want to consider the following studies if you're questioning, *Do I want lemon meringue pie or the Master Cleanse lemonade?*

Study One: University of Wisconsin–Madison. A group of rhesus monkeys were under observation since the mid-1980s at the University of Wisconsin–Madison. Half were randomly selected to eat as much as they desired for the rest of their lives, while the rest were on heavily restricted diets consisting of 30 percent fewer calories. Now, more than 25 years since the study first started, the researchers published their latest results. The control monkeys, which were on unrestricted diets, had roughly a three times greater risk of age-related death and disease than those that were calorie restricted. Of the 38 monkeys on each diet, 28 of the control monkeys died from age-related causes compared to just 10 in the restricted group. The diseases and disorders included diabetes, cancer, cardiovascular disease, brain atrophy, and bone loss, according to the study, which was published in the journal, *Nature Communications*. For all causes of death (including those not related to age), the control monkeys had a 1.8 times greater rate of death. In short, the monkeys consuming 30 percent fewer calories lived longer.

Study Two: The Salk Institute. In this study of round-worms at the Salk Institute, a critical gene that specifically links calorie restriction to longevity was identified. "After 72 years of not knowing how calorie restriction works, we finally have genetic evidence to unravel the underlying molecular program required for increased longevity in response to calorie restriction," reported Andrew Dillin, PhD, an associate professor in the Molecular and Cell Biology Laboratory. Dillin led the study, which was published in the May 2007 issue of the journal *Nature*. Currently it's the only strategy (apart from direct genetic manipulation) that consistently prolongs life and reduces the risk of cancer, diabetes, and cardiovascular disease. At the same time it wards off age-related neurodegeneration in laboratory animals, from mice to monkeys.

• •

No yo-yo: Don't regularly cycle on and off the MC. If you do, your body may end up lacking important nutrients. You'll also be more likely to set yourself up for long term weight gain!

• •

What Would My Doctor Probably Say?

Your physician may have some qualms because the Master Cleanse doesn't follow the standard American Dietetic Association's (ADA) recommended rules for weight loss. After all, you lose a lot of weight in a relatively short period of time. The ADA recommends losing, on average, only two pounds per week. Also, the MC doesn't recommend exercise during the 10-day program. That said, if you're generally healthy with no serious illness such as:

- diabetes,
- heart or kidney diseases,
- cancer,
- anemia,
- intestinal obstruction,
- gallstones,
- or are underweight or have a history of eating disorders,

the Master Cleanse done annually, biannually, or once every few months may be a winning program. If you're not sure whether you're a good candidate for the MC, definitely speak with your doctor to get the go-ahead.

Four Super-Power Ingredients

The recipe for the Master Cleanse only includes four ingredients: lemons, maple syrup, cayenne pepper, and water. Every one of these ingredients is packed with impressive healing properties.

Lemons

The ancient Egyptians believed drinking lemon juice could offer protection against several poisons. Well, they weren't far off. It's widely acknowledged today that lemons offer antibacterial, antiviral, and immune-boosting powers. Plus, they enhance weight loss because lemons are also a digestive aid and liver cleanser. In addition, lemons contain citric acid, calcium, magnesium, vitamin C, bioflavonoids, pectin, and limonene—all of which act to encourage immunity and fight infection. This little yellow fruit can:

- **Treat acne.** Because it contains citric acid, which contributes to our skin's glow. Lemons' alkalinity also kills some types of bacteria known to cause skin eruptions.
- **Help you de-stress and focus.** Research shows that lemon balm has a calming effect and therefore may be able to help reduce fatigue, exhaustion, dizziness, anxiety, nervousness, and tension. It's also believed that inhaling lemon oil helps to increase concentration and alertness.
- **Heal canker sores.** The antibacterial and antiviral properties found in lemons help to heal canker sores. One note of caution: There may be a burning sensation when the lemon juice comes into contact with your canker.
- **Ease colds.** When you have a cold, the healing power of lemons works both internally, by supplying

urgently required vitamin C to your defense cells, and externally, through the application of its antiviral properties on the mucous membranes in your mouth and throat.

- **Fight cholesterol.** The pectin in lemons, along with its other metabolic and circulation-boosting nutrients, can help lower cholesterol.

Cayenne Pepper

This hot pepper played a crucial role in Native American medicine and cuisine for thousands of years. It's also been used in traditional Chinese and Ayurvedic medicines for a variety of ailments. It can:

- **Calm irritation.** Cayenne has the ability to ease an upset stomach, ulcers, sore throats, and spasmodic and irritating coughs, as well as diarrhea.
- **Treat colds.** Because cayenne pepper works to break up and move congested mucus, it's effective in easing cold symptoms.
- **Fight fungus.** The results of one study indicate that cayenne pepper can effectively prevent the formation of the fungal pathogens phomopsis and collectotrichum.
- **Aid digestion.** Cayenne has been shown to stimulate the digestive tract and increase the flow of enzyme production and gastric juices. This aids the body's ability to metabolize food and eliminate toxins. Cayenne pepper is also helpful for relieving intestinal gas because it stimulates intestinal peristaltic motion, aiding in both assimilation and elimination.

- **Increase saliva.** Cayenne stimulates the production of saliva, which is important for optimal digestion as well as the maintenance of oral health.
- **Promote detoxing.** Since cayenne is a known circulatory stimulant, it also increases the pulse of the lymphatic and digestive rhythms. By heating the body, the natural process of detoxification is given a boost. Cayenne also causes us to sweat, another important process during detoxification.
- **Relieve joint pain.** Packed with a substance called capsaicin, when a cayenne pepper pack is applied to the area it acts to cause temporary heat on the skin, which sends chemical messengers from the skin into the joint, offering relief for joint pain.
- **Support weight loss.** Scientists at Quebec's Laval University found that participants who ate cayenne pepper for breakfast were found to have less appetite, leading to less caloric intake throughout the day. Cayenne is also a great metabolic booster, aiding the body in burning excess amounts of fats.
- **Help the heart.** This pepper has been shown to normalize blood pressure levels, as well as balance the body's low-density lipoprotein (LDL) cholesterol and triglycerides.

Some Like It Hot!

Cayenne is sold in several heat units. If you don't usually eat spicy foods, get the 30,000-heat-unit cayenne. If you're hot to trot, opt for higher units like African bird pepper, which is 80,000 heat units.

Water

If you think water is just about quenching your thirst, think again. Water is the very foundation of our lives. In fact, up to 60 percent of our bodies are made of water. H_2O will:

- **Boost metabolism.** Drinking water can boost your body's ability to burn fat. A study published in the *Journal of Clinical Endocrinology and Metabolism* found that drinking water increases metabolic rate by 30 percent in healthy men and women.

- **Fight hunger pangs.** Studies suggest that drinking one or two glasses of water before a meal can fill you up so you naturally eat less. And keep in mind, even mild dehydration will slow down metabolism by as much as 3 percent.

- **Protect the heart.** According to a six-year study published in the *American Journal of Epidemiology*, drinking water can lower your risk of heart attack. The research found that people who drank more than five glasses of water a day were 41 percent less likely to die from heart attacks during the study period than those who drank less than two glasses.

- **Ward off headaches.** In one study published in the journal *Neurology*, scientists recruited migraine sufferers and divided them into two groups: one took a placebo, the others were told to drink 1.5 liters of water (about six cups) in addition to their usual daily intake. At the end of two weeks, the water group had experienced 21 fewer hours of pain than those in the placebo group, as well as a decrease in pain intensity.

- **Boost brainpower.** Research shows that a dehydration level of just 1 percent of your body weight reduces thinking functions. On the flip side, drinking 8 to 10 cups of water per day can improve your levels of cognitive performance by as much as 30 percent.
- **Heighten attention.** Dehydration is the single most common cause of daytime fatigue. In fact, just a 2 percent dehydration level can trigger short-term memory problems and difficulty focusing on a computer screen or printed page.

Maple Syrup

This natural sweetener contains several properties that point to real health benefits. But like any sugar product (and maple syrup *is* sugar) it should be used strictly as advised. Opt for darker grades (B is the darkest) because they contain the most health-giving antioxidants. Maple syrup can:

- **Reduce inflammation.** It contains polyphenols, which are antioxidants that have been shown to quell inflammation, according to research from the University of Rhode Island. Inflammation is linked to several negative health problems, including arthritis and cancer.
- **Limit bloating.** Maple syrup is less likely to cause indigestion, gas, and bloating, compared with processed sweeteners.
- **Stifle sniffles.** Maple syrup contains essential nutrients like zinc and manganese, which can help

you ward off colds, according to a study conducted at Wayne State University in Detroit. And zinc keeps your level of white blood cells up, which is crucial for increasing your resistance to sickness.

. . . .

Nix vitamin and mineral supplements while on the Master Cleanse! Vitamins and minerals are provided during your Master Cleanse. Trying to add additional ones on your own can interfere with the detoxification process and reduce the effectiveness of the cleanse.

. . . .

Are You an Emotional Eater?

If you're an emotional eater, distinguishing between the real hunger pangs you'll feel at the start of the Master Cleanse with cravings to satisfy a deeper internal need may be a challenge. How do you know if you're an emotional eater? If you answer yes to any of these questions, it's a good indication that you are:

- Do you go for second helpings when you're feeling stressed?
- Do you eat even when you're no longer hungry or when you're feeling stuffed?
- Do you eat when you're feeling anxious, bored, angry, or sad to help you feel better?
- Do you use food as a way to reward yourself?

- Do you think food is your friend—maybe your best friend?
- Do you feel weak or out of control when you're around food?
  Here are some alternatives to emotional eating:
- If you're feeling depressed or lonely, call a positive friend who knows how to make you feel better. If you have a pet, now is a good time to connect with your four-legged friend.
- If you're feeling anxious, go for a long walk and allow your nervous energy to dissolve a little more with each stride.
- If you're feeling fatigued, take a warm bath, wrap yourself in a blanket, and allow yourself to enjoy a 20-minute nap.
- If you're feeling bored, read a page-tuner, catch up on an engaging hobby, or simply watch an amusing comedy.

Quiz: How Ready Are You for the Master Cleanse?

Before moving on to the next chapter, take this brief questionnaire to find out how prepared you are to partake in the 10-day Master Cleanse. Depending on your personal score, a corresponding analysis offers quick tips to boost your cleanse readiness.

1. When I imagine going on the Master Cleanse:
   a. It feels as if I'll be making huge sacrifices.
   b. I'm sure it will present some real challenges but will be a good jump-start to a healthier lifestyle.
   c. For the most part, I'm super excited! I've done these kinds of cleanses before and have a fair idea of what to expect.

2. On average, how much time do you have to devote to YOU:
   a. Between my relationships, work, and other responsibilities, probably not much more than a New York minute!
   b. I have to make the time—but I can do it. I know how to set priorities.
   c. I'm totally free from any real hassles over the next two weeks.

3. When I imagine meditating, it feels like:

  a. A real luxury. How can I make time to quiet my super-busy mind? I have so much I have to think about and need to do!

  b. Something I can accomplish. I've often thought about starting a meditation practice before.

  c. It's second nature. It's already part of my daily routine.

4. How do you deal with feelings of hunger?

  a. Honestly? I turn into a monster! I get "hangry."

  b. Okay. I mean it doesn't make me happy, but I can usually get through it.

  c. I don't mind the feeling. In fact, I sometimes find it pleasurable.

5. I'm going on the Master Cleanse because:

  a. My partner or doctor is getting on my case to radically change my eating habits and lifestyle.

  b. I want to lose weight and detox at the same time.

  c. This is the kind of health-promoting program that appeals to me on every level.

Scoring

Mostly A's: You need to wait another few weeks.

It's a better idea to begin the Master Cleanse when you have the time, mindset, and support from friends and family. If this isn't your situation right now, wait a few weeks so you can set yourself up to succeed. Here's what you can do in the meantime to prepare:

- Mark it on your calendar three to four weeks from today. It's good to have a goal!

- Give your family and friends notice about your plan and request their support. Try to avoid anyone who reacts with negativity.
- Post this affirmation on your fridge or mirror: I CAN AND *WILL* DO IT!

Mostly B's: You're almost there.

You've probably been thinking about going on some kind of detox cleanse or diet for a while now and you're just about ready to do it! Before blending the concoction and beginning the Master Cleanse, be sure to follow the preparation suggestions in the upcoming chapters. Give yourself an extra week to:

- Get off caffeine, sugar, and processed foods.
- Write down what you want to accomplish from the MC.
- Take care of any outstanding tasks or responsibilities in advance.

Mostly C's: You're ready!

You've done cleanses before so you know that even though it might not always be easy—or even enjoyable—it's so worth it! Since your physical being, as well as your emotional and spiritual life, are in balance, you'll probably only need a couple of days before beginning the regimen. To make the most of the Master Cleanse:

- Choose the best starting date. Are weekends or weekdays best to embark on the MC?
- Give away any food that might spoil during the 10 days you're on the MC.
- Let your friends, family, and colleagues know the dates of your cleanse.

• • • • • • • • • • • •

three

getting ready

Before anything else, preparation is the key to success.

—ALEXANDER GRAHAM BELL

You might be on the starting line poised to begin the Master Cleanse. Or, maybe you're hesitant, a little anxious, and unable to make a move. Either way this chapter will help you lean into the direction of the cleanse, gather your strength, and if you need it, bolster your confidence. What's the secret? Preparation. You'll learn easy-to-follow tips that can help you pave a smooth road so you'll be more likely to stay on course for the full 10 days without giving in to common obstacles, temptations, and sometimes unpleasant side effects. For those who were ready to begin five minutes ago, keep in mind that most valuable things in life are worth waiting for and working toward. The Master Cleanse is one of them.

Before the Cleanse

Before you begin your cleansing regimen, it's a good idea to allow yourself at least one week to prepare mentally, physically, and emotionally. If your score in the previous chapter's quiz showed the Master Cleanse might be more challenging for you, then heed the advice in the analysis and leave yourself an extra three to eight days to prepare and ease more gently into the detox.

Pre-MC Diet

For at least one week prior to the MC, reduce or eliminate:
- Caffeinated drinks such as coffee and tea
- Dehydrating liquids like alcohol and carbonated soda
- Processed foods
- Sugar
- Refined starches like bread and pasta
- Meat, poultry, and fish
- Dairy
- Supplements or vitamin pills

• •

No thanks, honey! Burroughs described honey as "predigested bee vomit" popular only among "gullible health foodists."

• •

Enjoy:
- Herbal tea or warm water with lemon
- At least six 8-ounce glasses of filtered water each day

- Plenty of salads
- Fresh fruits
- Sautéed root vegetables
- Seeds and nuts
- Clear soups like miso or vegetable broth
- Fresh virgin oil, coconut oils, spice, and lemon to flavor meals

Treatments

Sweeten life with a sauna. There are several studies showing saunas work to remove all kinds of toxins from your system, including solvents, PCBs, pharmaceuticals, and heavy metals that tend to hang out in our fat cells. Saunas also clear out about one-third of the toxic material that your kidneys work to remove from your bloodstream. Plus, there are benefits beyond detoxification. For example, the sauna's high temps invigorate your immune system; the number of white blood cells that fight infection increases as much as 58 percent the hotter you get in a sauna. Your T cells (which are also part of your immune system and antibodies) can increase by as much as 2,000 percent. Increased temperatures also help your body to secrete endorphins, which are those "feel good" chemicals in your brain. Endorphins make great painkillers, too. That's why folks suffering from chronic and acute pain can experience relief while sitting in a sauna.

Want more? Saunas can also help with weight loss. When you sweat heavily and flush the toxins out of your fat cells, it allows them to reduce in size, which can be helpful for dropping those unwanted pounds.

Experience a body scrub. Your skin is the largest organ of your body, and as you learned earlier (page 29), it plays a vital role in detoxification. A body scrub will stimulate your lymph and blood circulation through massage and also remove impurities from under your skin's surface. Typically, a body scrub has larger exfoliating particles than a facial scrub because the skin on your body isn't as delicate. Common ingredients in store-bought scrubs are salt, sugar, and crushed nut shells. If you buy a scrub, or go to a spa for a treatment, make sure there are no chemical exfoliants in it like alpha hydroxy and glycolic acids or salicylic acid, which can help improve the appearance of blemishes or redness but also end up putting toxins into your system.

You can make your own buffing scrub with natural ingredients like olive oil, honey, raw sugar, ground cloves, oatmeal, and even ground coffee. Adding your favorite essential oils to the mixture transforms your shower into an aromatherapy session.

• •

Make Your Own Sweet Body Scrub

> 15 drops vanilla essential oil or 1 teaspoon vanilla extract
>
> 1 cup fine brown sugar
>
> approximately ⅓ cup sweet patchouli, almond, vanilla, or other carrier oil (a carrier oil is a vegetable oil derived from the fatty portion of a plant, usually from the seeds, kernels, or nuts)

In a glass bowl, add essential oil or vanilla to sugar and stir thoroughly. Add almond or other oil gradually, stirring continuously. When the scrub is the consistency of sand it's ready to use.

• •

Relax with a lymphatic drainage massage. Your lymph system is a mega detox machine. It's made up of lymphatic vessels, lymph nodes, lymph (the interstitial fluid drained through the vessels), and lymphocytes (specialized immune cells). Your tonsils, adenoids, spleen, and thymus are also part of it. Your lymph nodes are soft, small internal structures located in your armpits, groin, and neck, as well as in the center of your chest and abdomen. They make your immune cells that fight infection. If your lymph cells are working well, they're simultaneously filtering lymph fluid to remove foreign material from your body. When bacteria or other immune threats are present in the lymphatic system, the nodes increase production of infection-fighting white blood cells, which can cause the nodes to swell. Most of us have had "swollen glands" at some time in our lives.

But here's the glitch: Your lymphatic system doesn't have a pump the way your circulatory system uses your heart. Instead it travels along when you move and breathe. If you don't get much exercise, breathe shallowly, or eat a lot of processed foods, the lymphatic system can become overtaxed, resulting in a susceptibility to infection and disease. That's where a lymphatic drainage massage comes in and why it can be so helpful to have one before you start your Master Cleanse.

A lymphatic drainage massage is a gentle style of bodywork that imitates the movement of your lymph vessels. Peripheral lymph vessels contract at a rate of 6 to 10 contractions per minute, so massage movements are repeated at the same slow rate. There's a rich bed of lymph capillaries right below your skin, and that's why it isn't necessary for a massage therapist to use much pressure to crank it up. An experienced masseur will use a light touch. Lymph fluid is drained toward lymph nodes in the neck, armpits, and groin before traveling to the largest lymph vessels and back into your cardiovascular system. A trained therapist will massage your lymph nodes first, and then work lymph toward the lymph nodes, before massaging your trunk and extremities.

Before booking an appointment, make sure you're going to see a licensed massage professional, ideally one who specializes in lymphatic drainage.

Do-It-Yourself Lymph Massage in the Shower

For the best at-home results, use a soapy sponge while you take a shower and enjoy 5 to 10 gentle repetitions on each lymph area:

- Begin by sponging from your neck to your collarbones. Then move down your chest and sponge in opposite circular motions.
- Next, move down to your abdomen and sponge in clockwise circular motions.
- For your legs and thighs, start by sponging from your feet to your hip socket in light upward strokes. Then, spend several minutes making clockwise circles on your thighs and up your gluteal muscles and hips.
- For your arms, stroke from your hands up to your shoulders, and make several clockwise circles around your upper arms.
- After your shower, towel dry and rest for at least 15 minutes.

Favor your feet with reflexology. This technique is a branch of complementary and alternative medicine that not only relieves stress but also targets problem areas in your body. Reflexologists, who are trained in offering this method, apply pressure to specific points on the feet (or hands), while you experience relaxation, increased circulation, and nerve transmission to the corresponding body systems. Reflexology may be used to stimulate specific areas, such as the heart, as well as the detoxing organs, specifically your kidneys, liver, and small intestine. Although it's not quite as relaxing, or perhaps as effective, as when you have a professional reflexologist offer a treatment, you can do it yourself.

For example, you can stimulate your small intestine, which is responsible for 90 percent of your digestion and absorption of food (the other 10 percent takes place in your stomach and large intestine). Thus, the main function of the small intestine is the absorption of nutrients and minerals from food. This self-reflexology exercise is especially helpful to do before you begin your MC.

Do-It-Yourself Reflexology

Step 1: Sit comfortably. The chair's seat should not elevate your knees above your hips. Both feet should be planted on the floor.

Step 2: Place a golf ball under the arch of your left foot. Slowly push your foot forward, which will force the golf ball to roll back toward your heel. Stop when the ball is resting just past your arch, in the indented space prior to the outward curve of the heel. You've just placed the ball on your small intestine point.

Step 3: Press down on the golf ball with your left foot until you feel pressure or slight discomfort, but not pain. Release the pressure by lifting your foot slightly and repeat as long as you can tolerate it.

Step 4: Next, switch feet and do the same thing on the right side. Remember, the small intestine pressure point is just beyond your main arch but before your heel curve.

Roll the ball from the tips of your toes to your heel to activate more pressure points.

Get a Reiki Treatment. This is a Japanese healing technique that can restore the flow of your body's energy through the placement of a professional practitioner's hands. A Reiki practitioner is trained in accessing powerful, healing energy, called Reiki energy. More and more westerners have been turning to this practice, which is often performed at complementary and alternative medicine centers. There have been studies that show its effectiveness. A 2010 study published in the *Research in Gerontological Nursing* journal looked at the effects of Reiki in the treatment of depression, anxiety, and other emotional issues. All 20 participants experienced some sort of positive response to the treatment, including a lower blood pressure and heart rate.

Exercise. When you're on the Master Cleanse, you will *not* be engaging in any strenuous activity. That's right! No pumping, spinning, running, jumping, Zumba, or strenuous yoga. In fact, it's a good idea to totally tone down working out a week before you're planning on going on the MC.

But, if you have a strenuous exercise routine, don't stop abruptly. Instead, opt for some gentle substitutions. You don't want to go through "exercise withdrawal." Research shows that when individuals who engage in regular physical activity abruptly stop exercising for even one week, they experience negative mood changes, especially feelings of fatigue, loss of vigor, and increased tension. After withdrawal from exercise for two weeks, participants in a 2006 study conducted at Uniformed Services of the Health Sciences in Bethesda, Maryland, felt further fatigued and experienced symptoms of depression and guilt.

Here are some easy-breezy exercise suggestions that can substitute for your more intense workouts. Feel free to choose your own, just make sure they aren't strenuous. No cheating!

- Strolling
- Fishing
- Light gardening
- Tai chi
- Restorative yoga poses

Try light therapy. This technique is most commonly used to treat seasonal affective disorder (SAD) by exposure to artificial light. SAD is a type of depression that occurs at a certain time each year, usually in the fall or winter. That said, light therapy can boost anybody's mood, anytime of the year. During light therapy, you sit or work near a device called a light therapy box. The box gives off bright light that mimics natural outdoor light. Light therapy is thought to affect brain chemicals linked to mood, easing SAD symptoms. Using a light therapy box may also help with other types of depression, sleep disorders, and other conditions.

Go Shopping

Since you won't have much energy to burn while you're on the MC and might prefer to stay in a meditative place, it's recommended that you shop for all the cleanse ingredients before you begin your regimen. Here's what you'll need:

- 60 to 80 medium-sized lemons (best if they're organic)
- 2 quarts of maple syrup (best if it's organic and Grade B, which is darker, grittier, thicker, more robust, and

has more minerals because it is produced later in the season)
- ½ cup of sea salt
- 10 gallons of filtered water, more if you want to drink it both as water and as tea
- 2 ounces of cayenne pepper (organic, if possible)
- Herbal laxative (Since you won't be getting adequate amounts of fiber during your cleansing period, it's necessary to take an herbal laxative to ensure that your colon functions and your body's wastes can be loosened and dislodged from your digestive system. Smooth Move, Senna, and Swiss Kriss are some popular commercial brands.)

••

Important! Stock up on toilet paper!

••

The Most Common Master Cleanse Mistakes

One of the best preparations any one can make before embarking on any adventure is to be aware of pitfalls. How else can you avoid them? Here are the biggest mistakes that most who people attempt the Master Cleanse fall for:

Not easing into the cleanse. If you don't prepare properly by slowly eliminating foods and reducing your hectic schedule, the detox side effects are likely to be more dramatic. You can find directions for what needs to be eliminated from your diet earlier in this chapter.

Not drinking all the lemonade. As you can tell by the shopping list, you'll be drinking *a lot* of lemonade—between 64 and 80 ounces *every* day. Although you can cut down on the amount of cayenne pepper (if you don't like it quite so hot) you must consume all the liquid.

Not following instructions. You might be tempted to purchase nonorganic lemons or drink from the tap instead of using filtered water, but that would mean you'll be introducing toxins into your system. Go for the gold and buy organic and filtered water.

Not doing the laxative or saltwater flush. You'll read more about these in the next chapter, and though they may not be pleasant, they need to be done. While the lemonade loosens toxins from your colon, the laxative and saltwater flush push it out for good. Go for it!

Not simplifying your schedule. It's very difficult to stay on this cleanse if you're trying to live your usual hectic life. During the first few days of the cleanse you'll probably need to be within a very short walking distance of a bathroom. Note: Give yourself at least 90 minutes after the morning saltwater flush before leaving your house.

Quiz: Test Your MC Know-How

Choose the answer you think is correct.

1. Who invented the Master Cleanse?
   a. Stanley Burroughs
   b. Robert Atkins

2. The foods you should eliminate at least one week before beginning the cleanse include:
   a. Coffee, tea, and other caffeinated beverages
   b. Nuts and seeds

3. Never substitute honey instead of maple syrup:
   a. True
   b. False

4. A sauna can:
   a. Boost your immune system and increase your heart rate
   b. Lower your blood pressure and increase your energy

5. Give yourself a week before you start the cleanse to:
   a. Unwind, relax, and ease out of strenuous workout routines
   b. Bump up your exercise routine to get your heart strong

6. How many organic lemons should you buy?
   a. 60 to 80
   b. 20 to 50

7. **What's the best grade of maple syrup to use?**
   a. Grade B
   b. Grade A

8. **A recommended exercise a week before the cleanse is:**
   a. Going for a walk
   b. Biking

9. **If you're in really good shape and you eat a healthy diet, you still need a week to tweak your diet and prepare for the MC.**
   a. True
   b. False

10. **How much filtered water will you need?**
    a. 10 gallons
    b. 5 gallons

11. **If you skip the herbal laxative you'll be sabotaging the plan:**
    a. True
    b. False

12. **The average weight loss after the MC is complete is:**
    a. 5 to 10 pounds
    b. 15 to 20 pounds

Scoring

Give Yourself 5 Points for all A answers, 0 for B answers

Between 50 and 60 points: You know your stuff!

You're a Cleanse Master (or Mistress)! You've either read the material carefully or you're already familiar with the basics of detox cleansing. Perhaps you've done one or more Master Cleanses before? In any case, there's no need for you to reread any parts of the book. If you'd like, move ahead now to the next chapter. After your week-long preparation is complete, you can begin the Master Cleanse. You are ready to change your life!

Between 30 and 45 points: You could use another quick look.

This score means that you may have missed some important information. Rather than race to the next chapter, it will serve you well to look over your score, note those areas where you had the wrong answer, and review the sections of the book you might have misunderstood or passed over. In order to successfully complete the cleanse, you'll want to know the facts. Knowledge really does help you through the cleanse. When you know what to do and why, as well as how it's benefiting your body, you'll likely be spurred on to successfully complete the 10-day course.

Below 25 points: You would benefit from a careful review.

Maybe you weren't paying much attention thus far, or you're not really committed to the cleanse so you skipped some sections. Take a moment now to set your intention. A simple affirmation such as "I want to complete the 10-day Master Cleanse" will help you get there. Once the commitment is set in your heart, go back and reread the book. You might also want to underline those areas that you missed or didn't understand the first time. When you're through, retake the quiz. There's an excellent chance you'll score high. Once you get those good results, you'll be ready to move on to the next chapter with the knowledge you need to succeed.

•••••••••••

four

starting the master cleanse

Everyone can perform magic, everyone can reach his goals, if he is able to think, if he is able to wait, if he is able to fast.

—HERMANN HESSE

Hopefully, you're feeling eager and ready emotionally and physically to give your life a big boost. If so, what are you waiting for? Let's begin the Master Cleanse!

The Night Before: Get Lax

The evening prior to beginning your Master Cleanse—and every evening while you're on the cleanse—you need to prepare your body by drinking one cup of a colon-moving drink such as Smooth Move Tea or Swiss Kriss. You can buy either one of these natural herbal laxative preparations at most health food stores. Directions are simple and on the box. Both require steeping the "tea leaves" in hot water and then sipping a full cup.

Why take a laxative? Well, when you're not eating, you're not getting enough fiber, which most of us know by now is a total must-have for peristalsis, the process that causes food to move through our digestive systems. That's why while you're on the Master Cleanse you have to use an herbal laxative to make sure your colon functions and causes the waste to be loosened and dislodged from your digestive system. Make "Detox, baby, detox," your mantra!

••

Don't get *too* lax! In general, you should never take laxatives on a long-term basis. Overuse is a big no-no. It can contribute to health problems (especially nutrient deficiency) or hide symptoms that may be from a serious medical condition (like colon cancer). If you're really into laxatives and end up relying on them, your bowel could become dependent on them and lose its lovely natural ability to eliminate on its own accord.

••

Guzzle the Saltwater Flush—*Before* the Lemonade Drink

In the morning, before you mix and drink your first glass of Master Cleanse lemonade, you'll also need to imbibe the once-daily saltwater flush (SWF). It's simple to make:

- 1 quart (32 fl oz) of filtered water (room temperature)
- 2 teaspoons sea salt

Stir until the salt is dissolved. Drink all of it within 10 minutes. So, why a SWF?

Because a SWF bypasses your bloodstream and works to flush your colon of the "debris" that will be loosened by the lemonade and laxative tea. That's why.

SWF Do's

- Use a straw to drink your 32 ounces of water. This puts the liquid at the back of your mouth when it hits and makes it so you don't have to taste it all the way down.
- Warm the water up a bit to help you get it down!
- Think of the lemonade mix from the Master Cleanse as a chaser.

SWF Don'ts

- Mix a small amount of water with the salt, then "chase" it with the rest of the water to mix in your stomach. This can cause hypertension as the salt will sit in your stomach for too long and disperse instead of using the weight of the water to push it through the body quickly.
- Put the salt in a tablet and then swallow with the water to "mix" in the stomach. Again, the salt must bond with the water prior to entering the body so that the weight pushes it through the body.
- Take a teaspoon of salt on a spoon and then swallow the full 32 ounces. Again, the important part of the

flush is that the salt and water must bond *before* ingestion. This is how the water weighs more. If taking them separately worked you could simply eat a salty diet and accomplish the same goal, which, as you know, doesn't work.

....

Really important! Stay close to a bathroom 60 to 90 minutes after drinking the SWF. There's a reason it's called a *flush!*

....

Countdown

Wait one full hour after drinking the SWF before preparing and drinking the MC lemonade.

Even though I mentioned some of these points in the previous chapter, they're super important to the success of your cleanse and worth reviewing before you prepare the lemonade drink and begin your Master Cleanse. Take heed:

- **The lemon juice must be fresh-squeezed.** This cannot be emphasized enough. It is necessary to use fresh produce. Bottled juice won't work and will erase most of the benefits of using the Master Cleanse diet.
- **The maple syrup must be 100 percent real, preferably Grade B.** It should not be the corn syrup–filled fake substitute.
- **The cayenne pepper is actually very important.** The cayenne pepper might seem unnecessary, but it helps to break up mucus and increases healthy blood flow. And to boot, it adds a bit of a kick.

The Master Cleanse Recipe

The Master Cleanse lemonade is prepared by thoroughly mixing these ingredients:

- 2 tablespoons freshly squeezed lemon juice. Lemon zest and pulp can be added if the lemons are organic and not artificially colored or treated with pesticides.
- 2 tablespoons maple syrup. Opt for the darker Grade B, which has more nutrients. If possible, buy organic syrup.
- $\frac{1}{10}$ teaspoon cayenne pepper (organic, if possible).
- 8 ounces filtered water.

Each day, drink a minimum of six 10-ounce glasses of the lemonade.

On the go? Prepare a day's supply in advance. Here's what you'll need:

- 1 gallon jug (a glass one is best)
- 10 fresh lemons, preferably organic
- Cayenne pepper powder
- Grade B maple syrup (organic, if possible)
- Measuring spoons
- Distilled water

Step 1: Fill the gallon jug halfway with distilled water.

Clean your gallon jug before filling it halfway with fresh, distilled water. This will leave room for your ingredients.

Step 2: Squeeze the fresh lemons.

Use your juicer or hand-squeeze fresh, unrefrigerated lemons. You will need 8 to 10 medium-sized lemons to provide the accurate amount of juice for a gallon of Master

Cleanse lemonade. After juicing the fresh lemons, measure 2 cups (32 tablespoons) of lemon juice. Add the lemon juice to the water.

Step 3: Add the maple syrup.

Add 2 cups of Grade B maple syrup into your gallon mixture.

Step 4: Mix cayenne pepper into your drink.

Measure 1 ½ to 2 teaspoons of cayenne pepper powder and add it to your mixture. Remember, cayenne stimulates digestion and increases blood flow in the body. Using cayenne gives the mixture a spicy edge, so try not to overseason.

Step 5: Shake! Shake! Shake!

Once you add all the ingredients to the gallon jug, fill it to the top with the rest of your distilled water. Firmly place the lid on it and then shake the mixture. You can refrigerate the concoction between uses. But remember to shake the jug prior to each use. The gallon jug will hold 128 ounces of your Master Cleanse mixture, which equals sixteen 8-ounce glasses.

Do It!

Drink one 8-ounce glass now.

Not bad, right? At last, you're on your way to experiencing a profound cleanse. Yay!

Important! Use all of the mixture prior to making more of the concoction in the same jug for the upcoming days.

MC Do's

- Drink your laxative tea at the same time each evening, preferably at least an hour before bedtime.
- Drink plenty of water throughout the day—every day. You need water to make sure you don't face dehydration.
- Focus on cleansing your body of toxins, and weight loss will come naturally.

MC Don't's

- Engage in strenuous workouts. The MC is about ending erratic, unhealthy eating, and rebooting and resetting your metabolism. This is much easier to do when you give your body a brief break from hyper-exercise. Trying to do heavy-duty workouts while following a limited caloric plan can create unwanted side effects, because the cleanse won't provide the extra fuel needed for exercise, or the added raw materials required for healing and recovery. As a result, doing both can leave you feeling tired, dizzy, and nauseous. It can also result in breaking down muscle mass, which can up your injury risk and lower your metabolic rate, the exact opposite of what you're aiming for.
- Use the MC as a way to purge. Emotionally using the MC (or any cleanse or detox program) as a method of purging so you undo the effects of bingeing is a big mistake. If you've found yourself on this roller coaster ride, reach out for help. All-or-nothing relationships with food are common for a lot of people, but they

aren't good for you physically or emotionally. Your ultimate goal is to strike a sustainable, healthy balance.

- Stay on the Master Cleanse longer than the recommended period.

Count to Three

For most people, after three days on the cleanse the program gets much easier—I promise. You'll probably begin to experience the benefits of clarity, calm, and concentrated energy. But to be honest, the first few days can feel like hunger hell. To put a lid on your appetite, you may want to try the following tips.

Five Ways to Slay Monster Cravings

Gain knowledge. It gives your gut power. The feeling of hunger is the first effect to kick in once you stop eating. Depending on what and how much you ate prior to the cleanse, it may take anywhere between an hour and half a day before your stomach starts to growl. The key to tackling this problem is *knowing* that the feelings of hunger will come and go during the MC. About 18 hours into the fast, a serious hunger manifests. This is the point at which the temptation to break the MC is usually at its greatest. However, when you force yourself to pull through, the hunger subsides after a few hours. By day three, it's likely to feel like smooth sailing. Honestly.

Be Zen about it. Hunger and getting hungry is something that we are taught to avoid. Try to allow yourself to experience the hunger without judging it as bad. Maybe just observe it and let the feeling pass. Make it more of a curiosity than a "bad" feeling. I'll even go as far as saying that you should embrace hunger and look forward to its benefits.

Guzzle water. Drinking an 8-ounce glass of water will blunt sensations of hunger within minutes. You may find that you are no longer hungry—or no longer *as* hungry—and can safely wait it out.

Stay engaged. One of the reasons it's so easy to fast overnight is because you're sleeping. When we're bored and not focused on something, we're more likely to be thinking about what our tummy is telling us. Read, watch a movie, play chess, meditate, paint, sew, write. Whatever you need to do to keep your mind off your stomach.

Take a trip down memory lane. When you feel like you just have to eat, remember how bloated some foods made you feel or how bad you felt in the past after overindulging. Recalling these icky feelings can instantly quell an appetite.

• •

"Disease, old age, and death are the result of accumulated poisons and congestion throughout the entire body."
—*Stanley Burroughs*

• •

Complementing the Master Cleanse

While you're cleansing you'll be open to inner expansiveness and change. So why not take this opportunity to work on detoxing and deepening your emotional and spiritual being? Vow to complement the Master Cleanse with restful, expansive inner work. Here are a few suggestions.

Practice Forgiveness

Don't kick yourself if you get annoyed every now and then. We all do that. But carrying a grudge is something else. Some scientists say if you're holding onto ill will your entire being suffers, including your body. On the other hand, learning to let go and open your heart can release stress and reduce pain and inflammation.

Here's why: Studies show stress exacerbates pain, tightens muscles, and interferes with the smooth running of the immune system—all things that have an effect on your health. It also interferes with a good night's sleep. Forgiveness turns it around. Research conducted by the University of Michigan's Institute for Social Research, Ann Arbor, reported that people who experience forgiveness had reduced levels of stress.

But most of us aren't saints and forgiveness may not come easily. Here are some techniques that can help:

- **If an apology is out there, try to accept it.** Allow someone the chance to apologize when they've hurt you. Letting someone apologize to you for the harm they have caused will help you to start healing and recognize that a situation was not their fault alone, or may not have been anyone's.
- **Realize that everyone makes mistakes.** We are all human and sometimes we are selfish people. Not

everyone means to be this way, but it happens. Try to think of the situation as a mistake.

- **Put it in perspective.** Understand that the resentment or anger you're feeling now happened in the past. It could be 30 minutes—or 30 years—ago.
- **Make a list of the upsides of the experience.** Chances are you've mulled over all the bad stuff again and again. Change your view. Make a list of 10 positive things that have come out of the experience.
- **Remember that a life well lived is your best revenge.** Stop focusing on wounded feelings—that gives the person who caused your pain power over you. Instead, look for the love, beauty, and kindness around you. And appreciate and embrace the family and friends who love you.

Grab Hold of Gratitude

Let's face it, sometimes it's really tough to experience gratitude, especially when we're struggling with difficult times. The cleanse may be one of those times because it not only brings up toxins in your body, but thoughts that are poisoning your mind and spirit. But gratitude is worth working on. Several studies have shown that a feeling of deep appreciation not only helps us deal with our problems but also helps to boost our health. Consider this: Researchers at the University of Connecticut found that patients who saw benefits and gains from their heart attack experienced a lower risk of having another one. Here are five simple ways to help you develop an attitude of gratitude:

- **Note all the good things in your life.** Even small events matter. For practice, keep a "good things" journal and write down all the wonderful things that happen to you during the day, from a child offering a smile to the sun shining. During times when it feels impossible to conjure up feelings of gratitude, open your journal and read through it for inspiration.
- **Hang out with positive people.** Optimism and feelings of gratitude are contagious. Likewise, if you surround yourself with negative people who are always complaining, it will be difficult for you to stay in an upbeat mood.
- **Be generous.** By giving to others, especially your time, your mind will focus on what you have rather than what you don't have. Unfortunately, most people focus on receiving, which only makes their mind focus on what they don't have. Research also shows that people who volunteer are generally happier—and live longer.
- **Write to someone who really matters.** Dr. Martin Seligman of the University of Pennsylvania recommends writing a 300-word letter to someone who changed your life for the better. Be specific about what the person did and how it affected you.
- **Be clear.** Don't confuse gratitude with indebtedness. Sure, you may feel obliged to return a favor, but that's not gratitude, at least not the way psychologists define it. Indebtedness is more of a negative feeling and doesn't yield the same benefits as gratitude, which inclines you to be nice to anyone, not just a benefactor.

Remember Your Dreams

Most of us wake after a compelling dream with a shadowy feeling there was deeper meaning behind our nocturnal wanderings. But how do we unlock its message? The first step is to remember everything we can. But it's estimated that only 3 to 10 percent of people can actually recall their dreams regularly. The rest of us? Not so much. If you want to remember your dreams, here's how to do it:

- **Give voice to your intention.** Just before sleep, voice out loud your desire to remember your dreams. Saying the words implants a stronger message in your brain.

- **Keep writing material within reach.** Place a journal dedicated to your dreams on your night table beside your bed. Also keep several pens and a flashlight right beside it. Date your dream journal entry before you fall asleep each night. This helps produce an expectation that you'll remember your dreams.

- **Set your alarm.** You want to wake at a specified point during the night. If you are worried about waking a partner, then drinking several large glasses of water prior to bed may be another way to assure you will awaken.

- **Keep a regular sleep routine.** This means starting your night of sleep in the same position every night, as well as going to bed and waking at the same time.

- **Awaken with questions.** Upon awakening, gently probe your mind and pay attention to bodily sensations. If you don't immediately remember your dreams, stay with a feeling and follow it by asking the feeling to be amplified. If you're in a different physical position than you were while dreaming, try shifting your body back into that position.

- **Write everything down.** Include all sensory impressions that come to mind: colors, images, sounds, tastes, people's expressions, settings, feelings, and emotions. Even though you are groggy and tired when waking, it's worth it to write as much as you can before you forget.

Go Slow

Studies show taking it slow is good for our health and well-being. It lowers inflammation, stabilizes blood pressure, keeps glucose levels steady, helps in decision making, and ultimately makes us happier. When you're cleansing, your body is giving you the message to slow down. Take heed! The following tips can help you to turn it down a few notches.

- **Give it a day.** Take an entire day when you make it your goal to be patient. At the end of it, write down all the ways it helped you. Like any skill, developing patience takes practice.
- **Breathe.** When you're frustrated and in a hurry, *stop*. Take several deep breaths. For example, if you're in heavy traffic, make the decision to pause and not get worked up. Remind yourself that getting impatient won't make things move along any faster, so why get worked up for nothing? Now breathe deeply.
- **Practice thinking before speaking.** When we're hurrying or letting emotions run wild, we often blurt out the first thought that comes into our heads. Next

time hold your tongue, consider what you want to say first, and think about the consequences. You can avoid hurting or offending others by slowing down reaction time.

- **Remind yourself some things take time.** Think about your happiest memories. Chances are, they were instances when your patience paid off, like when you worked steadily toward a goal that wasn't immediately gratifying, or took a little extra leisure time with a loved one. Would you have those memories if you had been impatient? Probably not. Good things may not always come to those who wait, but most good things that do come don't come right away.

- **Expect the unexpected.** Yes, you have plans, but things don't always work out as planned. Accept the twists and turns in life gracefully. Keep your expectations realistic. This applies not only to circumstances, but also the behavior of those around you.

Find Your Personal Power Boost

Now that you've started your journey on the Master Cleanse, you may discover that you'll meet negative obstacles, or goal-blockers, along the way. I call them my "inner naysayers"; another word is "demons." The good news is that you needn't give in to your naysayers because *you* have the power to defeat them. That said, it helps to know your strongest source of strength. The following quiz will help you zero in on your personal power.

QUIZ: Discover Your Strongest Suit and Overcome Obstacles

When the going gets tough each of us has a personal power that we draw on to help us succeed. It resides deep in our primal brain area, which is lodged in the subconscious, so we may not be aware of what gives us our special boost. Take this quiz to uncover your secret source of power—and make the most of it!

1. When packing for a trip, I usually:
    a. Give myself a small but comfortable margin of time to spare.
    b. Throw things into the suitcase at the last minute.
    c. Pack carefully and well in advance.

2. The last time I was stuck in traffic, I:
    a. Tuned into music and just kept inching my way along.
    b. Switched lanes to get ahead.
    c. Turned on the traffic report to get an idea of the delay.

3. When I make a mistake, I'm more likely to think:
    a. Let me try again.
    b. What can I learn from this?
    c. How can I do it differently next time?

4. Evenings are a great time to:
   a. Curl up in front of the TV.
   b. Catch up on whatever chores still need to get done.
   c. Plan tomorrow's schedule.

5. In high school my best subject was:
   a. English or history.
   b. Art or music.
   c. Math or science.

6. If a dish I plan to serve to guests doesn't come out as expected, I'm most likely to:
   a. Serve it with a smile anyway.
   b. Doctor it up—fast!
   c. Switch it up with a microwaved meal.

7. If I'm not sure whether I'm going out on the town after work, I'll:
   a. Wear something fancy for the day.
   b. Put on my best accessories to dress up a causal outfit.
   c. Take along a change of clothes.

8. When it comes to watching television, I usually:
   a. Go with my favorites.
   b. Channel surf.
   c. Check the listings in advance.

9. Would you consult a feng shui expert before redecorating and follow her advice?
   a. If it matched my decorating taste.
   b. Absolutely.
   c. Probably not.

10. If the forecast was for bright skies—but there were sudden looming clouds just as you were about to leave for a picnic—would you be more likely to:

   a. Take your chances and leave just as you are!
   b. Reschedule plans.
   c. Grab rain gear.

Scoring

Total your score.

Mostly A's: Your inner power comes from resiliency.

You bounce right back because you know making a mistake is just part of the process, a stepping stone toward your goal. You're deeply positive, optimistic, and self-confident. It's why you can keep walking forward no matter what difficulties you encounter. You know you'll succeed—and you're right! Studies show resiliency is the number one trait of folks who rank highest on the scale of emotional intelligence, a prime predictor of success. Since you believe the adage *one door closes, another opens*, you know any disappointments are just a blip on the screen.

Mostly B's: Your inner power comes from flexibility.

Outstanding at finding alternative routes to your goals, you're super adaptable, can change directions easily, and stay open-minded to a wide range of possibilities. In fact, change makes you *happy*. Folks who are flexible are excited about navigating around different directions. They consider difficulty a challenge—not a defeat. Spontaneous, able to think on your feet, and naturally creative, you have a real sense of adventure about life. And since you can bend easily, even when there's a sudden surprise and plans fall apart, you remain calm, steady, and centered.

Mostly C's: Your inner power comes from a strong sense of reason.

As a strategic thinker, you can analyze any situation and think through problems quickly. Your secret? You're able to look at both the big picture and small details all at once. You also know how to evaluate information. You gather advice and research the facts, but ultimately use your own sense of practical reasoning to come to the right conclusion. As someone who knows how to stand back *and* look ahead, you schedule your day, plan for the future, and stay organized and fully prepared—which means whatever life hands over, you're ready for it!

•••••••••••

five

what to
expect

We must learn to reawaken and keep ourselves
awake, not by mechanical aid, but by an infinite
expectation of the dawn.

—HENRY DAVID THOREAU

There's no way to get around it. If you want to reap all the
awesome benefits of the Master Cleanse, you need to stay
on it for 10 days—no less, no longer. I promise you this: it's
worth it. By Day 10 you'll awaken to a brand-new world. Ten
days is the time it takes your body to completely cleanse and
renew your organs. In 10 days you'll reset your entire being.
Keeping this in mind, does it surprise you to learn that the
number 10 also holds profound significance in other areas
of life besides detoxing? Well, read on!

Ponder the Power of 10

Mystics have always known the virtue of the number 10. In tarot cards, 10 is represented by the Wheel of Fortune and can be interpreted as forces that can help or hinder you suddenly or unpredictably. In the Kabbalah (the metaphysical system by which its students learn about God and the universe), 10 is the number said to be boundless in origin and having no ending. According to the Kabbalah, 10 also denotes a change in conditions and rules both the spiritual and scientific aspects of life. In astrology, 10 rules the planet Uranus and also signifies change. In numerology, the study of the occult significance of numbers, 10 means "all." It represents all sorts of new changes in life. Through the vibration of 10, numerologists also contend, you have the insight and power to recognize and understand the needs of humanity and the ability to bring peace and harmony to all. Ten resonates with the vibrations and energies of leadership, optimism, confidence, independence, creative powers, success, energy, originality, adaptability, determination, and individuality. Ten also represents beginning new lessons in the cycles of knowledge. With all this in mind, why doubt 10 days is the ideal time to be on the MC?

Detox Changes

During the 10 days and nights you're on the Master Cleanse, there will be plenty of highs and lows. You might want to write down the changes you're experiencing. Note not only your physical reactions, but also your mental, emotional, and spiritual insights. Of course, not everyone is the same, and that's why the experience can vary wildly. During this time, your body might kick your immune system into high gear and that's the reason for these experiences. Try to go with the flow when, and if, you have unpleasant reactions. It means your body is in the process of detoxing. But just to give you a heads-up as to what you might or might not experience, here's a guide to the side effects of the Master Cleanse. Be grateful if you experience any of the following side effects. It means you're detoxing!

Diarrhea. First ask yourself "Is it *really* diarrhea?" If you're having four or five watery bowel movements a day while you're on the MC, it's not diarrhea. Diarrhea is an all-day affair. The SWF only produces eliminations for 90 minutes after you drink it. If it really is diarrhea, you can stop the laxative and saltwater flush until the condition ends.

••

WARNING: If it's really diarrhea and it continues for more than three days, stop the cleanse! If it continues after that, see your healthcare practitioner.

••

Emotional highs and lows. Some people have total meltdowns, when they weep for days. Others have reported having a closer relationship to their spiritual selves. This may be the underlying reason why ancient cultures used fasts as a way to get closer to God or nature's power.

Hair loss. This happens rarely—but it happens. The good news? It's temporary. And it usually happens to people who do the Master Cleanse too frequently. It could be the result of an alkaline mineral (calcium, magnesium, and potassium) imbalance that can be remedied easily by taking supplements at the close of the Master Cleanse.

Tummy aches. Since there's less waste in your intestines, you might feel contractions or cramping. Honestly, they can be pretty uncomfortable. Hang in there. They can be dealt with by drinking more water or lemonade. This gives the intestines something to push—and they're made happy. This remedy should do the trick within minutes.

Caffeine withdrawal. If you consumed caffeine prior to the cleanse, your withdrawal will feel as severe as your addiction was. That's why it's suggested you stop using caffeine products before the MC starts!

Coated tongue. This is an indication of the effectiveness of the cleanse. Your somewhat nasty-looking tongue will become a lovely pink at the end of 10 days.

Cravings. You may crave certain foods, flavors, even cigarettes—even if you gave the habit up years ago! This is your body's way of informing you that a particular mucus layer is breaking up for removal. Do not give in to these cravings. The next day they'll be gone, thanks to the saltwater flush.

Other possible symptoms:
- Headache
- Stuffed or runny nose/congestion

- Sore throat and swollen glands
- Coughing and sneezing
- Fatigue, muscle aches, and other cold and flu symptoms
- Skin irritation, such as rashes and pimples
- Burning bowel movements (from the cayenne pepper)
- Irritability

Conventional medicine labels these symptoms Jarisch-Herxheimer Reactions. In alternative medicine, they're considered simply detox or healing effects. The detox process lets you know you're eliminating poisons. These effects may make you feel crummy temporarily, but ultimately, they'll help you feel great!

• •

When the going gets tough, remind yourself:
- I'll have more energy.
- My sleep will be deep and restorative.
- My skin will be super soft.
- I'll have lots more mental clarity.
- Pounds will drop!

• •

Day by Day

The Master Cleanse is not about willpower. It's about knowledge, knowing what to expect, and dealing with it effectively. There may be some variables, but for the most part, this is a general outline of daily experiences many people have while on the cleanse:

Day One isn't usually difficult. However, if you have a serious caffeine habit, you might be carrying around a headache for the first few days. The caffeine headache usually peaks before Day Four, and after that, it's generally clear sailing in the head department.

Days Two and Three may be the toughest. On the other hand, some folks just move along without a blip. During these first few days, your body will be burning muscle in order to gain energy. Keep in mind that no matter what you're feeling, like everything in life, it's not permanent and will pass. This is a time when irritability can take hold. It's a known symptom of detoxing. Boredom, anxiety, and the desire to chew something—*anything*—can be at the forefront of your thoughts.

Days Four to Six make up the time period when detoxers report lots of good stuff happening. It's the period when your body begins to burn fat and waste for energy. When this happens, most folks report feeling a new sense of calm, focus, positivity, and boost in energy. You might also note that you're starting to lose weight. Plus, your sense of smell will most likely be heightened.

Days Seven to Ten you might experience a detachment from food. It feels as though you can go on forever without eating a morsel. You might also discover you're no longer interested in watching television or reading the newspaper. There's a new sense of inner exploration that may bring you to a quieter, more reflective, and meditative place. This is a fine time to write your thoughts down in your journal. Dreams might also be more vivid. You may also notice that your skin feels clearer and your body more flexible, lithe, and at ease.

• •

Feeling chilled? No worries. It's cool. The cleanse lowers your metabolism, which naturally makes the body feel colder.

• •

What If You Don't Feel Any Detox Symptoms?

If you're not noticing any side effects, you may be wondering whether your body is actually detoxing. No worries! Continue on your Master Cleanse for the full 10 days. For example, even if the pounds aren't dropping, your body will be changing shape and you'll be losing inches. Also, some people have slow systems and find that once they end the Master Cleanse, they start to experience detox symptoms. Remember: it's a personal journey. This could be a sign that you had a low level of toxicity in your body. Or you might be missing some important element of the MC. Let's review. Are you:

- Drinking the saltwater flush every morning as quickly as possible?
- Mixing two tablespoons of fresh-squeezed (not bottled) lemon juice into each 10-ounce glass individually, or making only enough for a day's batch?
- Using at least 1/10 of a teaspoon of cayenne pepper, or if you are sensitive, gradually increasing the amount until you reach this level?
- Refraining from eating or drinking anything else?
- Were you constipated before the cleanse? This can slow down the results.

- Overweight? This, too, can mean you might need to wait a little longer before you experience the MC effects.

What If the Detox Symptoms Feel Way Over the Top?

The more toxicity in your system, the more difficult the first few days of the MC will be. This might be a result of emotional imbalance like anger, jealousy, or depression, or it could be the result of extra weight, medications, allergies, lots of environmental toxins in your system, an extremely bad diet, or booze. Whatever the reason, it will pass as you detox. The answer to your distress is to emphasize the elimination part of the Master Cleanse by only drinking six glasses of the lemonade, rather than 10. Be sure to continue with the saltwater flush as well as the laxative. It's also a good idea to take a nice warm bath in the early evening (for around 20 minutes) with two cups of Epsom salts diluted in the water. This helps you relax while giving the detox a boost.

However, if it really gets bad, you can always discontinue the Master Cleanse and attempt it at another time. Life gives you lots of chances to get healthy. It's a journey.

- Don't be hard on yourself.
- Don't judge yourself.
- Don't give up on future improvement.

In Praise of Your Colon

Your colon, also known as your large bowel or large intestine, is part of your digestive system (also called the digestive tract). Your digestive system is the group of organs that allows you to eat and use the food you eat to fuel your body with energy. Since lots of the detox actions take place through your colon, this organ is worthy of a more comprehensive understanding.

What Exactly Does Your Colon Do?

Your colon plays a huge role in how your body uses the food you consume. This is the journey food takes through your body, from start to finish:

Step One. Food begins in your mouth. Here it's chewed by your teeth into smaller pieces. At the same time, your salivary glands release juices (saliva) that help the food get softer and tinier. Your tongue, along with your saliva, turn the food into numerous itty-bitty pieces that are ready to slide into your esophagus. The esophagus is a 10-inch-long tube that connects to your stomach. Muscles in the esophagus move food into your stomach.

Step Two. While in your stomach, protein substances, or enzymes (also known as gastric juices), break down the food into ever smaller bits. Your stomach has mighty muscles that are able to churn up the food until it's a creamy liquid. This stuff moves into your small bowel.

Step Three. While in your small bowel, believe it or not, these food particles get even smaller. More juices (enzymes), this time from your pancreas, liver, and gallbladder, mix together in your small intestine. It's right here where all those crucial vitamins and nutrients move through the blood vessels that are in the lining of your small bowel. Then the blood takes the nutrients to other organs in the body. Nutrients are used to help repair cells and tissue.

Step Four. What's left over? Mostly liquid that moves into your colon. The water is absorbed in your colon while the bacteria in the colon break down the remaining material. Next, your colon moves the leftover material into the rectum.

Step Five. Your rectum is like a storage holder for waste. Muscles in the rectum move the waste, called stool, out of your body through the anus.

Why Is Your Colon So Important?

A healthy colon gets rid of the leftovers it no longer needs. Your stool is filled with bacteria, so it's super important to pass this out of your body. If your colon isn't working the way it should, you'll experience problems, which include bloating, gas, and pain.

Let's Talk Tongue

As mentioned before, your tongue will go through a transformation while you're on the Master Cleanse. That's because your tongue is a living barometer reflecting the level of your body's toxicity. The first few days on the cleanse your tongue might turn whitish, with a thick, gross coating. Don't despair! In a few days you'll begin to notice your tongue turning a lovely pink, starting around the edges; finally, the plaque will recede from the front of your tongue toward the back.

When the 10-day cleanse is over and moving forward, you might want to consider using a tongue scraper. This is a common practice in India, where the gunk on the tongue is considered toxic. In fact, there's some research to show that a tongue scraper is more effective at removing toxins and bacteria from the tongue than a toothbrush. And consider this: almost half of our oral bacteria live on in the deep crevices of our tongue. Scrapers are inexpensive, and you'll be able to buy one at most health food stores or online. The best is a stainless steel scraper because it's easiest to clean. You can always use the side of a stainless steel spoon until you get a tongue scraper. Need more convincing? Here's what else a tongue scraper does:

- **Banishes bad breath.** Most bad breath comes from the back of the tongue where a toothbrush has a tough time reaching. Tongue scraping significantly reduces and removes oral bacteria from the crevices of all areas of the tongue.
- **Enhances flavor.** Proper digestion begins with taste and salivation. If you don't take steps to remove toxic

mucus on the tongue, your taste buds can become blocked. Removing build-up from the surface of your tongue helps open pores and exposes your tender taste buds.

- **Boosts your immunity.** Tongue scraping prevents toxins from being reabsorbed into your body and boosts overall immune function.
- **Cuts cavities.** Scraping helps to remove bacteria and toxins that are responsible for periodontal problems, plaque build-up, tooth decay, loss of teeth, gum infections, and gum recession.
- **Improves digestion.** You know that proper digestion is considered to be the foundation of health. Hopefully, that's why you're on the MC. Scraping activates saliva production and promotes "agni" (the word in Ayurvedic medicine for your body's digestive fire) to help with digestion.

How to Scrape Your Tongue

While you're standing in front of a mirror, scrape your tongue by simply holding the two ends of the scraper in both hands, sticking out your tongue, and placing the scraper as far back on your tongue as possible. With firm but gentle pressure, scrape the surface of your tongue in one long stroke. Rinse the scraper and repeat until your tongue feels clean and is free of coating (usually 5 to 10 times).

IMPORTANT! Only begin this practice once your cleanse is over. Do not scrape while on the cleanse. Your tongue will divest itself of toxins during the course of the detox.

A Weighty Matter

Mostly everyone who stays on the Master Cleanse for 10 days and follows instructions will drop pounds, and *plenty*— as much as 20 pounds. And it's not just water weight. A good deal of it may be weighty fecal matter that's accumulated inside your body, sometimes for years. Of course, some of it is water weight, and you'll lose that, too. After all, the MC is essentially a fast. It does provide needed nutrients, but obviously it's not something you can maintain for a long period of time. Because of the fasting aspect, there will be some pretty drastic weight loss initially. Some folks are so surprised by the major weight loss that it frightens them into quitting the program early. Know this: the Master Cleanse will not cause you to lose an unhealthy amount of weight. Yes, you'll probably shed several pounds of fat, but who doesn't want that?

All this said, the MC is not designed to use as a weight loss diet. Its goal is to promote health and well-being on all levels—physical, spiritual, and emotional. When you use the Master Cleanse appropriately, it will help to wholly cleanse your systems. The best way to lose weight and maintain the loss you've managed is to eat a health-conscious diet every day when you're not on the cleanse.

Opening Your Heart

Cleansing is a tender time. It helps you be vulnerable, open, and ready to tap into deeper parts of yourself. I recommend you use this precious time to allow your beautiful heart chakra to open and radiate love and joy.

According to ancient teachings, humans possess seven major energy centers. These centers are called chakras and they radiate throughout the body, both side to side and front to back. In Sanskrit the word "chakra" means "wheel." So, imagine spinning wheels. The chakras start at the base of your spine and run all the way to the top of your head. Each chakra has a particular frequency vibration.

The center for unconditional love is located in the fourth chakra at the center of your chest. It's in charge of your heart and circulatory system, respiratory system, arms, shoulders, hands, diaphragm, ribs/breasts, and thymus gland. Lots of emotional issues such as love, grief, hatred, anger, jealousy, fears of betrayal and loneliness, as well as the ability to heal ourselves are located here, in our fourth chakra. From this position in the middle of the body, the fourth chakra is the balance between your body and spirit.

This chakra is the place where unconditional love is centered. Unconditional love is a creative and powerful energy that can guide and help us through the most difficult times, including those when inner strength is needed to continue on the cleansing path. This energy is available in any moment, if we turn our attention to it and use it to free us from our limits and fears.

Metta Practice

A powerful practice to open to and embody unconditional love is one from the Buddhist tradition. It is called Metta practice and only takes 15 minutes to do each day. I suggest you give it a try during your MC. Here's how:

- Sit in a comfy and relaxed manner. Take two or three deep breaths with slow, long, and complete exhalations. Let go of any concerns or preoccupations. For a few minutes, feel or imagine the breath moving through the center of your chest—in the area of your heart.
- Mentally repeat, slowly and steadily, the following or similar phrases:

    May I be happy.

    May I be well.

    May I be peaceful and at ease.
- While repeating these phrases let yourself experience the intentions they express. Loving-kindness meditation consists primarily of connecting to the intention of wishing ourselves or others happiness.
- After a period of directing loving-kindness toward yourself, bring to mind a friend or someone in your life who has deeply cared for you. Then slowly repeat phrases of loving-kindness toward them:

    May you be happy.

    May you be well.

    May you be peaceful and at ease.
- As you say these phrases, again sink into their intention or heartfelt meaning. And, if any feelings of loving-kindness arise, connect the feelings with the phrases so that the feelings may become stronger as you repeat the words.
- Sometimes during loving-kindness meditation, seemingly opposite feelings such as anger, grief, or sadness may arise. Take these to be signs that your

heart is softening, revealing what is held there. You can either shift to mindfulness practice or you can—with whatever patience, acceptance, and kindness you can muster for such feelings—direct loving kindness toward them.

Do not judge yourself for having negative feelings. Just see them and release them.

Okay, now that you know what to expect and have some understanding about the forces at play in your physical, psychic, and emotional being, it's a good time to call on your innate ability to see this adventure to its healthy conclusion.

You can help key in to your individual ability to meet challenges with this quiz.

Quiz: What's Your Innate Ability to Meet Challenges?

We all have an inborn mechanism that helps us manage challenges. Tuning in to key personality traits like the ability to look at the big picture, take advice, and be patient can help you overcome obstacles and successfully complete the Master Cleanse. Take this quiz to see whether you're inspired by challenge. Then get tips on how to make the most of what comes naturally to you.

1. **If a colleague were out sick and your boss put her work on your desk, you would:**
    a. Do what you could comfortably take on.
    b. Take care of it all, even if it meant staying late.

2. **The kind of vacation your prefer most is:**
    a. A lazy, relaxed holiday at a beach retreat.
    b. A trip to a new place, where there's lots to do and see.

3. **If your best friend offered to fix dinner, you would be more likely to:**
    a. Relax and enjoy the fruits of her labor.
    b. Express your appreciation and offer to pitch in.

4. **When you meet new people, you're more focused on:**
    a. Getting to know them.
    b. Making a good impression.

5. You typically wake up and:
   a. Jump out of bed, in a good mood and ready to tackle the day.
   b. Slowly stretch and ease into the new day.

6. What's your dream vacation for two?:
   a. Thrills and chills Disney World.
   b. Cross-country RV trip visiting far-flung relatives.

7. When you make a mistake you think:
   a. What can I learn from this?
   b. How can I correct it?

8. You sometimes forget your phone.
   a. True.
   b. False.

Scoring

Give yourself 10 points for each A answer and 5 points for each B answer.

Between 60 and 80 points: You're naturally easygoing.

You can let problems and projects flow in and out of your life while staying calm and collected because your *immediate* reaction is not to control, fix, or change them. Instead you process situations slowly, asking a lot of questions and weighing the pros and cons before coming to a conclusion. You'll also ask for support if you need it. Psychological studies on happiness show this approach will lead you to decisions that meld with what's truly best for you. The downside is others may view you as passive and in some cases you *do* take a backseat. After you gather all the facts, here's how to be more proactive:

- Ask yourself "How am I really feeling?" Let yourself experience negative emotions. Naturally easygoing people have a tendency to sugarcoat or repress their authentic reaction.
- Make a list of actions or goals you need to reach and then give yourself a deadline to achieve them. Take actions step by step so you don't feel overwhelmed.
- Become a leader. If you're coping with a situation that involves other people, trust yourself to be at the helm. Calm types like you can diffuse or mediate a situation effectively because you don't get emotionally charged.

Between 40 and 55 points: You're inspired by stress.

Whatever the task, you're determined to do it quickly and perfectly, leaving no stone unturned. "I can't" is just not in your vocabulary. This type of personality is actually turned on by difficulty and inspired by challenge. In fact, when there's a job to be done you go the extra mile to make sure it's done just right. Being an overachiever is admirable, but you may find yourself bored with routine—even creating extra work for yourself just to keep life interesting. What's more, since you want everything to go perfectly, it might be difficult to let go of control. With so many logs in the fire, burnout is also possible. So aim for balance. Here's how:

- Schedule pleasurable activities. Stress junkies have a hard time sitting still, so recharge by making stress-free but fun dates with friends and family.
- Delegate. Trust others who have expertise to carry some of the load. If you're feeling insecure, it's okay to check in once in a while.

- Open your palms. Surprisingly, a study shows this simple gesture of letting go actually helps release the impulse to take over.

35 points or less: You're sometimes overwhelmed.

Scoring within this range means you usually react to situations emotionally and often feel a little anxious, especially when new situations present themselves. You might have had a recent disappointment and that makes you wary of new situations. Add to the mix your busy schedule trying to balance work, family, and social responsibilities, and who wouldn't feel overwhelmed? No wonder you look for quick fixes! You don't have the time—or so you think—to dig deeper and come up with a more grounded approach. To avoid feeling overwhelmed, try these coping techniques:

- Get the emotion out first. Let yourself cry or yell. Or you might try a kickboxing class, writing in a journal, or viewing a comedy for a hearty belly laugh. As long as you get the emotion out first, the stress level will be reduced.
- Go on a mind vacation and allow your decisions to evolve. Window shop, take a walk, just loll around at home. We do our best problem solving subconsciously. Just by giving yourself time before taking action, your decisions will evolve from reactionary (or emotionally charged) to intuitive.
- Take action without expectation. Try not to label your decisions or work either a success or a failure. This approach will help you to continue to move along toward your goal without self-criticism.

- Check in again. Allow yourself to take another break if you start to feel overwhelmed. Signs include a head-ache, muscle tension, nail biting, difficulty breathing, or even clenching your jaw.

• • • • • • • • • • • •

You're on the detox adventure of a lifetime! When you're ready to exit the Master Cleanse, turn to the next chapter.

six

easing out of the cleanse

Everything has to come to an end, sometime.

—L. FRANK BAUM,
AUTHOR OF *THE WIZARD OF OZ*

Perhaps you've just completed 10 days of the Master Cleanse, and surprisingly, you now feel like staying on it a for a few more days. Yes, it happens! That's okay to do if, indeed, you have lots of experience with the cleanse and you've been through it at least a few times over the years, and have followed it from start to finish. But if you're a beginner, understand this is a restrictive cleanse which means that it's best done for a particular amount of time. *Ten days.* Staying on it for too long is just plain unhealthy. If this is your first experience with the MC, it's time to call it quits.

Your 10 Days Are Up

You may have ambivalence about ending the cleanse now because you're feeling so lithe and joyful and are no longer experiencing hunger or cravings. But all good things must come to an end. That said, don't exit your cleanse with a drastic change in diet. For example, don't consume a burger and fries—or even a bowl of tempeh. You've just put your body through major changes. Exiting the cleanse should be a conscious, slow, and careful process.

Here are important guidelines to follow:

Day One. Stick to drinking just liquids. Some folks like to continue with the lemonade drink for at least another day or two. As long as you're not also taking laxatives or drinking a SWF, that's fine. I recommend enjoying fresh-squeezed orange juice (preferably organic) along with lots of water (you may want to use it to dilute the juice). Don't gulp! Sip it slowly and let it settle blissfully in your belly. OJ is excellent in helping with the digestion of food, which, don't worry, will apply to you later. Besides, who knew orange juice could be so sweet and utterly delicious? Consider how the orange grows on the tree from its fragrant white blossom to a robust bright fruit. Think about how it relies on the sun for growth—and consider how we do, too.

Day Two. Continue drinking orange juice as well as plenty of water. Today you can add a vegetable broth (try vegetable bouillon cubes) or a light, homemade vegetable soup. (See recipe below.) If you're feeling desperate to chew on something crunchy, opt for gluten-free crackers. These foods are easy on the stomach and will help your digestive tract get back to work.

• •

Lovely and Light Veggie Soup

4 teaspoons olive oil

1 medium onion, medium diced

kosher salt and freshly ground black pepper, to taste

2 medium carrots, medium diced

2 garlic gloves, finely chopped

1 celery rib, medium diced

2 cups vegetables, medium diced (your choice, such as cabbage, asparagus, fennel, or peas)

1 quart low-sodium vegetable broth (made from bouillon cube)

Heat olive oil in a large saucepan over medium-high heat until crackling. Lower heat slightly. Add the onion, season with salt and pepper, and cook, stirring occasionally, until clear (about 5 minutes). Add carrots and garlic and cook for about 2 minutes, stirring occasionally. Add the celery and the hardier vegetables, such as cabbage and fennel. Cook an additional 7 minutes. Add any quicker-cooking vegetables, such as asparagus and peas. Add the broth and bring the soup to a boil, then reduce the heat to low. Gently simmer uncovered for about 15 minutes. Season to taste. Sip slowly while you ponder the ingredients and appreciate the taste sensations.

• •

Day Three. Today continue with the soup, OJ, and plenty of water, but for dinner you can add a fruit and steamed vegetables of your choice, washed down with several glasses of water.

Day Four and Beyond. Now you're ready to ease your body back to a regular eating plan. But watch your portions. As you begin to experience hunger and your cravings return, it may be tempting to pile your plate high. Psychologically, you may feel as if you "deserve" it after your "deprivation." But do your body a favor and don't rush it. One technique that helps is to choose a smaller-sized plate. Another is to be sure to chew all your food slowly and mindfully. It's also a good idea to avoid meat and dairy for a few more days. Both these foods are difficult to digest. In fact, if it's possible, avoid meat for at least a couple of weeks after the fast.

Eat Breakfast

Research shows that breakfast eaters typically consume about 100 fewer calories during the course of the day and weigh less than those who don't eat in the morning. Approximately 80 percent of participants in the National Weight Control Registry (which charts dieters who have kept off 30 pounds for a year or longer) have breakfast every day. What's an added benefit to eating a nutrient-dense morning meal? It supplies glucose to your brain, which helps you think clearly and function optimally until lunchtime.

How to Keep the Pounds Off

While certain foods can push our appetite button and encourage us to continue consuming (think salty chips), scientists have found that certain flavors can put a damper on our cravings. The following five foods are among the most potent appetite suppressants:

Vegetable juice. Loaded with fiber and plenty of water thanks to ingredients like celery and watermelon, this drink is considered a "high-volume" food. In one study, participants who drank vegetable juice before a meal ended up taking in 135 fewer calories. It's best to make your own, but you can also buy store-bought varieties as long as they have low sodium. Check the label.

Dark chocolate. Great news! Researchers in Copenhagen found that the intense flavor of dark chocolate makes you feel full. The label needs to read 70 percent cocoa content. Note: Milk chocolate consists of both cocoa butter and butter fat, a combination that makes you digest your food faster. In any case, you'll need to practice portion control. Two pieces tops.

Hot sauce. Not only will this add full flavor to your meals, but thanks to the ingredient capsaicin (found in chile peppers), which triggers the appetite-suppressing hormone, leptin, you're likely to eat less. You don't have to wait for a burrito, either. Be creative. You can spice up anything, from eggs to eggplant.

Almonds. These nuts are not only rich in vitamin E, magnesium, and antioxidants, they can help control your appetite by stabilizing your blood sugar levels and making you feel full. It takes about half an hour for the almonds' appetite-reducing effect to kick in, so have a few before you start to feel famished. Since nuts are fattening, eat no more than a handful a day.

Apples. A terrific source of fiber, apples also work to suppress your appetite by expanding your stomach and helping you to feel full. Apples also act by keeping your blood sugar levels consistent so you don't experience a "sugar crash" that triggers cravings. Plus, apples require lots of chewing time, which helps slow you down and gives your body more time to realize that you're no longer hungry. Caveat: Buy organic apples. The others are loaded with pesticides.

How to Stay Chill and Relaxed

When stressed to the max it's not unusual to crave salty, sweet, and processed foods. But that kind of diet only adds to feelings of anxiety. If you substitute unhealthy cravings for smart choices, you can calm your nerves and stay cool as a cucumber. To reduce stress and anxiety, try these six power foods.

Nuts. Research shows a connection between selenium deficiency and increased anxiety, depression, and fatigue. (Selenium is a mineral that's been shown to have beneficial effects on metabolic function.) You can turn it around by eating nuts (particularly Brazil nuts). Just a handful a day does the trick. Other sources of selenium include shitake mushrooms, tuna, cod, and salmon.

Spinach. Popeye's snack of choice contains heaps of magnesium, which helps to keep your nerves steady and your muscles in a relaxed state. Your body will let you know if you don't have enough magnesium, not only by pumping up your anxiety, but with muscle tension, cramps, and fatigue. Try to include one cup of fresh spinach or half a cup of cooked spinach to your diet each day.

Dark chocolate. The amino acid tryptophan is essential in helping the body to create serotonin, a neurochemical that eases anxiety. Lucky us—dark chocolate is rich in tryptophan! Other foods that contain tryptophan include sunflower seeds, sesame seeds, nuts, legumes, and dark turkey.

Herbs. Opt for basil, an excellent source of magnesium that helps muscles and blood vessels to relax. Bonus: It also contains antibacterial and anti-inflammatory properties that are useful if you have rheumatoid arthritis or inflammatory bowel conditions. Other calming herbs include lemon balm and chamomile, both of which you can drink in a tea.

Oats. Complex carbohydrates enhance the absorption of tryptophan, which is in turn used to manufacture serotonin. To get the soothing effect from oats, eat them together with some proteins such as nuts or seeds. Or, opt for brown rice, unrefined grains, or legumes.

Broccoli. Rich in potassium and beta-carotene, as well as vitamins C and E, broccoli not only gives your immune system a boost but is the perfect food to relax your nerves. Other sources of potassium include avocado, banana, kale, brussels sprouts, cabbage, winter squash, eggplant, and tomatoes.

How to Keep Your Post-Fast, Youthful Glow

Certain foods have the ability to work against the natural aging process and fight disease while doing it. If you want to turn back the hands of time, consider adding these eight power foods to your diet.

Garlic. All members of the allium family (which includes onions, chives, leeks, and shallots) contain sulfur compounds that research shows can protect blood vessels and help prevent heart attacks and stroke. Plus, studies also show that these compounds have cancer-fighting properties.

Asparagus. This green vegetable not only naturally detoxes your body but also works as a diuretic. The secret is in the fiber-filled stalks. Asparagus also contains inulin, a prebiotic that helps those probiotics already in your digestive tract to flourish. Asparagus are also a major source of vitamins and minerals.

Watermelon. The zinc in watermelon cleanses toxins from the body, especially from the bladder and kidneys. And since 90 percent of watermelon is water, it quenches thirst, fills you up, and makes you eat less. This natural anti-aging food contains vitamins A, B, C, and E; minerals zinc and selenium; and essential fats.

Basil. This herb has the ability to reduce and hold back inflammation. The best way to eat basil is raw since the power of the plant's oils are lessened by the drying process. FYI: The same benefits hold true for mint.

Avocado. An excellent source of antioxidants, fiber, vitamins C and K, and folate, avocados are also one of the best sources of the monounsaturated fat oleic acid. What's the big deal? Oleic acid lowers LDL, or so-called bad, cholesterol.

Dark berries. Both blueberries and blackberries give the heart, brain, and skin a big boost. The secret is anthocyanin, the flavonoid that gives these berries their color. Just make sure to go organic, if possible, since most berries, if grown conventionally, contain high levels of pesticide.

Coffee. Yes! You've given this up for the cleanse but you might consider retriggering that caffeine habit. Why? Because this wake-me-up brew is loaded with antioxidants that studies show can not only improve concentration, but memory, as well. But more than one or two cups a day can make you feel anxious. So don't overdo it.

Green tea. Just like coffee, green tea contains caffeine that boosts memory and concentration, but it has even more benefits. Studies show it can boost immunity, suppress appetite, and lower blood pressure. Researchers at the University of Basel, Switzerland found that people who drank green tea had greater activity in the working-memory area of their brains.

••

Foods to Avoid Eating at Night

Who doesn't get the nighttime munchies? Even if it's just an answer to the occasional craving, certain "bad" foods can wreak havoc on your body and particularly your sleep cycle if eaten in the evening. Here are the worst offenders:

Red meat. This is double trouble. First, if the meat is a fatty cut such as a rib eye steak, it will take a long time to digest and your stomach will remain active while you're ready to call it a day. Second, red meat contains an amino acid called tyrosine, which triggers brain activity.

Pizza. Loaded with carbs, not to mention cheese, sauce, meat, and whatever other toppings you choose, a pie can really kick your metabolism around. All that fat mixed with the acid from the tomato sauce and grease is a recipe for acid reflux.

Ice cream. This tempting food is a top choice for late-night nibblers, but most brands contain lots of sugar. In fact, any sugary dessert will make your blood sugar level soar and then drop rapidly. If you opt for chocolate or coffee ice cream, you'll up the chance of staying awake since they both contain caffeine, which revs you up when you need to calm down.

Cereals. Ever wonder why it's called a "breakfast cereal"? Shaking out a bowlful is a quick appetite fix but it won't help you sleep. Most commercial brands contain heaps of sugar. If you like to have cereal at night, read the label carefully and choose one that's low in sugar and high in fiber. The mixture of carbs and fiber will help you fall asleep instead of keep you awake.

Chips and salsa. If you're in the mood for something spicy, you may reach for the classic pairing of chips and salsa. However, the spiciness of the salsa can trigger acid reflux. Combine that with carb-filled chips and your stomach could be partying throughout the night.

Garlic bread. It's not only the carbs that will keep you awake. Garlic (a healthy ingredient earlier in the day), like other spicy foods, contains compounds that cause heartburn and acid reflux.

Pasta. Pasta is simply carbohydrates, and these kinds of starches will affect your blood sugar level, making it difficult to fall asleep. Pasta, along with the oil, cheese, and heavy sauce, is a combination that turns to fat, especially if eaten right before bedtime.

Beyond Your Appetite

Halt Negative Thinking

A big bugaboo when it comes to reaping the benefits of the Master Cleanse is allowing negative thinking to seep back into your daily life. In the same way that you can consciously choose not to allow unhealthy foods to return to your daily diet, you can pay attention to your thoughts and consciously choose to ban negative and self-defeating thoughts from reentering your mind.

Negative thoughts drain you of energy and keep you from being in the present moment. The more you give in to self-defeating thoughts, the stronger their energy becomes. Even a tiny naysaying thought can snowball into an avalanche of negativity. On the other hand, a positive thought can manifest into a vast universe of possibility.

Here are six ways to stop negative thinking from taking up valuable real estate in your head.

- **Smile.** When you smile you actually increase mood-boosting endorphins.
- **Watch your language.** Instead of saying "This is too hard" or "I'll never be able to stick to healthy foods," substitute with "This is a challenge!" and "I'll keep trying!"
- **Help someone.** Volunteering can provide a healthy boost to your self-confidence, self-esteem, and life satisfaction. You are doing good for others and the community, which provides a natural sense of accomplishment. Your role as a volunteer can also

give you a sense of pride and identity. And the better you feel about yourself, the more likely you are to have a positive view of your life and future goals.

- **Forgive yourself.** If you slip up, it's not a biggie. Remind yourself no one is perfect all the time because we're human. We all make mistakes. Don't dwell—let it go!

- **Make a list of five reasons you're grateful.** Being grateful helps you appreciate what you already have and what you've already accomplished. If you have more reasons, go for it.

- **Post positive quotes from folks you respect.** These are two of my faves:

> "Believe that life is worth living and your belief will help create the fact."
>
> —William James

or

> "Once you replace negative thoughts with positive ones, you'll start having positive results."
>
> —Willie Nelson

Get Your Mojo Working

During the 10-day cleanse you've taken a hiatus from strenuous exercising. Now you can reintroduce more taxing physical activity into your daily life. It's a good idea to start slowly with moderate workouts. Here are some suggestions.

Walking. Maybe you've been going for slow walks during your cleanse. Well, now you can bump up the speed a bit. One hour of moderately paced walking can burn about

250 or more calories and give you a decent cardiovascular workout. A word of caution: If you haven't moved much at all during the cleanse, or you're feeling a little weak, it's best to start walking about 10 to 15 minutes at a time and slowly increase your time by about five-minute intervals to allow the cardiovascular system and muscles time to adapt to the new demands.

Swimming. Water is a fantastic medium for low-impact exercise. This is especially true when the water's warm, ranging between 83 and 88 degrees Fahrenheit. Submerging the body in warm water increases the body's temperature, which also increases circulation. One of the reasons water provides a healthy place to exercise after a cleanse is that its buoyancy removes much of the weight off your joints and muscles that haven't been very active during these 10 days. Water also adds resistance for your extremities, helping build strength. Water exercise options include swimming laps, walking in place in deep water, or water aerobics classes. FYI: A hot tub can be a therapeutic way to massage aggravated muscles and relax after a workout.

Tai chi. This Chinese system of exercises dates back thousands of years. It's practiced through a series of slow-moving poses originally designed for self defense, mental calm, and lucidity through its graceful circular movements and breathing techniques. Though the effects of tai chi lack much scientific study, it is believed to increase flexibility, strengthen muscles, develop balance, and improve range of motion while keeping the mind clear and focused. If you don't have a tai chi practice, post-cleanse is a perfect time to begin because you'll feel more open to possibilities and your ability to focus will be heightened.

Yoga. If you're one of the three people left in the United States who don't have a yoga practice, post-cleanse is an ideal time to begin. "Yoga" literally means "to unite or yoke." The practice unites movement and breath and can help ease stiffness and tension in muscles and joints, as well as zoom in on a meditative mind and deep breathing. If you already have a yoga practice, for the first week after the cleanse, concentrate on restorative poses like child's pose and pigeon. If you're a newbie, let your instructor know that you're just coming off the Master Cleanse and need to take it particularly slow and easy. One of the great things about yoga is that poses can be adjusted to fit your particular needs.

Biking. This is a great way to feel the wind in your hair and at the same time get in a low-impact aerobic exercise that improves the strength of your heart, hips, and knees. If it's winter, cycling can be done indoors on a stationary bike. If cycling is new to you, start with short time slots of at least 10 minutes. Then extend those as your stamina improves. If you're a seasoned cyclist, now is *not* the time to go to a spin class. Give yourself at least two weeks to return to your pre-cleanse stamina.

Quiz: Are You Nice Enough to Yourself?

Surveys show the number one complaint most Americans have is that they don't have enough time for themselves. After the Master Cleanse, continue being good to yourself. This is crucial to maintaining your physical health and emotional well-being. Being good to yourself doesn't mean you're being selfish or egotistical or not caring for those you love; it means you value your life and all the gifts it presents to you. Take this test to discover whether you need just a touch (or lots) more TLC—and get tips on easy ways you can get what you deserve.

1. Which would matter *most* when purchasing a new sofa?
   a. How durable it is.
   b. How it will look in my living room.
   c. How it feels when I sit on it.

2. When someone makes me angry, I usually:
   a. Breathe deeply to release the feelings, but keep it to myself.
   b. Simmer for a while, then later explain what upset me.
   c. Vent quickly—loudly—then forget about it.

3. I read for sheer pleasure:
   a. Rarely.
   b. Sometimes.
   c. Frequently.

4. In family photos, I'm usually:
   a. Not there since I'm the one who thought to bring the camera.
   b. Wherever there's an open spot.
   c. Smiling center stage.

5. How many items are usually on your to-do list?
   a. At least six.
   b. A few high-priority must-dos.
   c. What list?

6. The last time I was drawn to buying a new article of clothing, I:
   a. Used my willpower and passed it up.
   b. Considered carefully before buying it.
   c. Grabbed it.

7. When I'm on vacation for more than a week, I:
   a. Worry about everything I'm *not* doing.
   b. Wonder about everyone back home.
   c. Thank my lucky stars every day for the break!

8. Aside from my keys and handbag, the item I would make sure to have before heading out is my:
   a. Watch.
   b. Cell phone.
   c. Book or iPod.

9. If there were no eggs for the family's Sunday breakfast, I would be more likely to:
   a. Go right to the store, without checking myself first in the mirror.
   b. Wash my face, comb my hair, and then go.
   c. Pour cereal instead.

10. When I have a day to myself, I usually spend it:

a. Catching up on chores.

b. Mellowing out with a hobby or watching TV.

c. With family or friends.

11. When hosting a party I can be found:

a. Making sure every last detail is perfect.

b. Introducing guests to one another, and helping them feel comfortable.

c. Just enjoying myself.

12. How often do you sit down for three meals a day?

a. Rarely.

b. Often.

c. Always.

13. When I'm dealing with a problem, I'm more likely to:

a. Work it out by myself.

b. Seek advice from an expert.

c. Ask family and close friends for their help.

Scoring

Mostly A'S: You could use some TLC.

Always running at top speed, you give 110 percent of yourself to everything you do. And while you get an occasional self-indulged moment, you tend to allow virtually everyone—and everything—to take priority over your own needs. This sort of selflessness can leave you feeling depleted on every level. The solution? Recharge with special time all to yourself. Try:

- Setting aside 15 minutes of "me" time each day. "Journal keeping, reading, or 'soul' strolls are all effective ways to recharge your spirit," says Al Siebert,

PhD, author of *The Resiliency Advantage: Master Change, Thrive under Pressure, and Bounce Back from Setbacks*.

- Learning to say *no*. This isn't easy for most women. So, begin with small compromises. For example, instead of organizing the entire hospital or office party, agree to be in charge of drinks or the cake.
- Treating you. Whether it's a pampering massage, a day at the beach, or an indulgent movie matinee, remember you deserve a reward.

Mostly B's: Your needs are usually met.

Basically you know how to strike an even balance between your responsibilities and personal needs. But there are times when your good deeds or tireless efforts go unnoticed, and naturally, you feel disappointment. Eventually, this can lead to a wall of resentment that drains your energy. Here are some ways to get the credit you deserve:

- Speak up. Taking credit for a job well done will help you feel your effort was worth it.
- Opt for a hiatus. See how quickly others appreciate your selfless habits once you take a break from your boundless good deeds.
- Learn to simply say "thank you" whenever you get compliments. Siebert says, "Studies show people who can accept compliments easily get almost twice as many as those who are too modest."

Mostly C'S: You're your own best friend.

You intuitively understand that to be good to others you need to be good to yourself. That's why you've learned to put your own peace of mind first, overlook the small stuff, and still make time for others. You've also learned to accept the praise you deserve without feeling uncomfortable. And when there's a break in your schedule you jump at the chance to pamper yourself. But don't stop there. Here are ways to give you an *instant* lift even when time is super tight.

- Buy a bunch of flowers. Studies show just looking at a flower arrangement will raise your level of feel-good endorphins.
- Gaze at the sky. Staring at moving clouds for just a few minutes can unleash muscle tension.
- Wear something yellow. "Yellow makes you feel good about yourself and the world," says Leatrice Eiseman, author of *Colors for Your Every Mood*.

•••••••••••

More Ways to Keep Yourself Happy

Look at an aquarium. Studies going back as far as the late '80s have shown that gazing at an aquarium reduces stress and subsequently lowers blood pressure. Researchers have compared the effects of hypnosis vs. an aquarium, fishless vs. fish-filled aquariums, and no aquarium vs. having an aquarium. In all cases, viewing some sort of aquarium reduced blood pressure and promoted feelings of well-being. Even watching a video tape of fish has been proven to have therapeutic effects.

Use petal power. Flowers might be the perfect pick-me-up if you don't consider yourself a "happy morning person." Participants of a behavioral study conducted by researchers at Harvard University and Massachusetts General Hospital confirmed that they feel least positive in the early hours, but reported being happier and more energetic after looking at flowers first thing in the morning.

Opt for a view. Hospital patients who were assigned to rooms with a pleasant outdoor view recovered faster from an operation and were discharged sooner than those looking at a brick wall. The theory is that if a good view helps patients recover, it must surely help the rest of us keep healthy by lifting our moods, easing stress, and providing a deep sense of optimism. If the view from your window isn't expansive, try surrounding yourself with pictures or photos of favorite places.

Take a whiff. "Specific odors can trigger vivid memories and nostalgic feelings—and if the memories they evoke are pleasant ones, they'll lower your stress level and improve your mood," says Alan Hirsch, MD, assistant professor of neurology and psychiatry at Rush-Presbyterian-St. Luke's Medical Center in Chicago. Some favorite mood-boosters: Play-Doh, peppermint, freshly baked apples, and vanilla.

Chew gum. This was a no-no while you were on the cleanse but it might make you feel good now. During tests to recall 15 words, gum-chewers remembered two to three more than the non-chewers. The reason? According to Andrew Scholey of the University of Northumbria in Newcastle, UK, chewing gum helped deliver more oxygen and glucose to the brain, not only increasing concentration but also boosting overall mood and confidence.

Be a dancing queen. Whether you cha-cha-cha, break dance, hip-hop, or polka, according to Mayo Clinic researchers, you're not only improving your muscle tone and coordination, but dancing your way to increased energy, reduced stress, and lowered blood pressure.

LOL. Watch a sitcom or stand-up comedy show, read the comics, find jokes online, or hang out with a funny friend, and you'll find yourself in a good mood. Research confirms laughter reduces the level of stress hormones like cortisol and epinephrine. Plus, it increases the level of health-enhancing hormones like endorphins and neurotransmitters. What's more, a hearty ha-ha-ha increases the number of antibody-producing cells and enhances the effectiveness of T cells. All this means a stronger immune system, as well as fewer physical effects of stress. FYI: Even fake laughter can deliver some anti-stress hormones.

Pet a furry friend. Pet owners tend to visit their doctors less often and are less likely to suffer from depression. But if you don't own a pet, it's no problem. Stroking or being near friendly animals can also lower heart rates and reduce blood pressure levels; so for happiness benefits, visit a pet store or volunteer at your local humane society.

Surround yourself in silence. Noise creates a type of chronic stress that puts the body into a state of raised alert. Even when you're asleep, your body continues to react to sounds, pumping out stress hormones. These can cause changes to the heart and blood vessels that contribute to high blood pressure, heart attacks, and stroke. To make yourself happy and relaxed, create a quiet sanctuary in your own home. If that's not possible, visit your local library, house of worship, or a peaceful spot in a public park.

Stand tall. There's something to be said for our mother's admonitions to stand straight. The *Wall Street Journal* reports that according to a German study, participants who were standing in an upright position (compared with those whose postures were bent) wrote more original and uplifting stories when shown pictures open to personal interpretation. Poor posture also puts strain on muscles, tendons, and ligaments, wearing out the joints and even affecting the efficiency of internal organs.

Now that you have the tools you can use to keep your mind and emotional life in shape, turn to the next chapter to sample recipes for yummy, super-healthy meals and snacks.

seven

keeping your diet detoxed

Tell me what you eat, and I will tell you who you are.

—BRILLAT-SAVARIN,
AUTHOR OF *THE CELEBRATED BOOK ON
GASTRONOMY, THE PHYSIOLOGY OF TASTE*

You look and feel fabulous and you're sleeping like a stone. Right? So, how do you hold onto your state of superlative well-being for the following weeks and months to come? The best way to do it is to change your eating habits, especially if your diet was extremely toxic before the cleanse. Many people go on the MC in the first place because they've been consuming lots of unhealthy foods. If that's you, don't look back! Look ahead and begin anew. The MC kickstarted you to a new level of eating, thinking, and feeling. You've stopped eating all those foods that cause allergies, sensitivities, and inflammation. Now is your opportunity to transition to a healthy eating plan that's permanent.

Your new diet should be filled with all the good stuff—fruits, vegetables, fermented soy (like tempeh and miso), whole grains, and small, carefully chosen amounts of dairy. But you'll be avoiding the yucky stuff like gluten, sugar, and most dairy. By steering away from these ingredients, and keeping your mind in a stress-free zone, you should be able to continue feeling almost as great as you did right after you completed the Master Cleanse.

Hold Onto Your Good Health

It's important enough to repeat: When you begin to reintroduce foods, don't do it all at once. Start slowly with small portions. The reentry process takes some patience, but it's important to go easy to avoid the return of digestive problems.

Some foods are notorious for causing crummy reactions post-MC. Here's a list of the four most common culprits to *avoid*:

Wheat. Gluten has the biggest impact. Folks claim to have more energy, fewer digestive problems, and less food cravings when they permanently eliminate gluten from their diets. If you "cheat" and eat gluten-rich foods, you may experience noticeable discomfort.

How to Tell If You're Allergic to Gluten

If you're one of the estimated 10 percent of Americans who is sensitive to the protein found in wheat, rye, and barley, you might be gluten intolerant. And if the ingredient isn't limited or removed entirely from your diet, and you develop a full-blown allergy, it could cause damage to your small intestine. Here are some signs of gluten intolerance:

Headaches. While there's no specific type of headache associated with gluten intolerance, it usually comes on within 30 minutes to an hour after eating gluten.

Exhaustion after eating. Most of us can feel a dip in our energy after eating a big meal while our body is metabolizing the food. But how about just a sandwich? Take note if you feel wiped out after consuming even small amounts of gluten.

Sensation in extremities. If you experience joint pain, numbness, or tingling in your arms and legs after eating gluten, it's an indication of intolerance.

Mood changes. If there's a significant shift in your emotional state after eating wheat, rye, or barley, that's another sign. Most specifically, those with the condition complain of feeling suddenly irritable or anxious.

Confusion. The inability to focus is another common complaint. Do you easily lose your train of thought and find it difficult to concentrate after consuming gluten?

Weight changes. Gluten sensitivities are most notably associated with weight loss, but gluten intolerance can also result in unexplained weight gain over time.

Sugar. You may notice your sugar cravings have gone away. That's the addictive nature of sugar; when you have a little bit you want more. When you don't have any, you don't need it. Here are some reasons why you should give up sugar:

- *It's addictive.* Just like a drug, sugar stimulates the release of dopamine, a "feel-good" chemical in the brain. The more sugar you consume, the more your body creates dopamine receptors that lead you to crave more sugar. It's a vicious cycle of increasing sugar consumption.
- *It hurts the immune system.* For hours after consuming sugar, the efficiency of white blood cells goes down, hindering your immune system and the ability to fight disease and infection.
- *It steals minerals.* Sugar has absolutely no nutritional value (although plenty of empty calories), which is bad enough, but it also robs the body of essential minerals like sodium, potassium, magnesium, and calcium. This can weaken the teeth and bones, causing tooth decay and diseases like osteoporosis.
- *Sugar is bad for your liver.* Refined sugar is half glucose and half fructose. The liver is the only organ that can metabolize fructose. When too much fructose enters the liver, it gets turned into fat that can build up over time and ultimately lead to disease.
- *It causes weight gain and diabetes.* Insulin drives glucose into cells from the bloodstream. Elevated

blood glucose is toxic, so when excessive amounts of glucose cannot be used properly, the pancreas begins to secrete insulin in order to remove it from the bloodstream, leading the body to become insulin-resistant. When the body becomes resistant to insulin, the pancreas stops doing its job properly, which is a contributing factor to type 2 diabetes. Insulin also signals the body to store fat, which leads to obesity.

• *It adds years.* Sugar ages you because it can attach to proteins in the bloodstream, resulting in Advanced Glycation End Products (AGEs) that damage collagen and elastin production, which are responsible for maintaining skin's elasticity.

• *It makes you emotionally unstable.* Sugar can lead to depression, anxiety, chronic fatigue, irritability, and mood swings. That's because sugar leads to a spike in both blood sugar and feel-good serotonin levels in the brain. When the sugar withdraws from our system, we experience a "crash," creating a cycle of craving and bingeing in both our bodies and our minds.

• *It affects your cholesterol.* High sugar consumption lowers levels of the "good" high-density lipoprotein (HDL) cholesterol that helps remove LDL, or "bad" cholesterol from the artery walls, and has been shown to increase levels of triglycerides, a type of fat found in the blood that poses an increased risk for heart disease.

• *Don't opt for the fake stuff.* Artificial sweeteners, while not made from sugar, should also be avoided at all costs. These sweeteners are made from loads of chemicals with absolutely no nutritional value and a slew of harmful side effects of their own.

Too much dairy. Avoiding dairy usually helps if you have digestive problems, skin issues, congestion, sinus problems, or allergies. People who are able to tolerate having some goat cheese, sheep's feta, or buffalo mozzarella do better staying away from cow products. Some people are able to have yogurt, but can't have any milk. You can experiment and see what works best for you.

Strawberries. I know, bummer. But people who have been on the MC report being highly sensitive to strawberries after the cleanse. If you're a real strawberry lover, try a couple. If you experience a scratchy throat when you start eating them again, avoid strawberries for at least another month.

So, what can you eat? Lots! Read on for recipe ideas.

eight

revelatory recipes

The key to holding onto all the amazing benefits you've gained through the Master Cleanse is to allow your body to transition into eating healthful meals that require minimal digestive effort but offer maximum taste and satisfaction.

You'll be offered several recipe choices for each of your three major meals—breakfast, lunch, and dinner—as well as various nutritious snacks and a few dessert choices. It's worth repeating that overeating is a big no-no, so even though the recipes are often for more than one individual, either share with your family, invite guests over (socializing is the best spice to add to a meal!), or store leftovers in a tightly sealed container and reheat—preferably not in a microwave.

In any case, always use fresh ingredients when possible and remember to eat slowly and consciously.

Bon appétit!

Kitchen Staples

When the cupboards are bare, we're more likely to dash out of the house and grab whatever we see first. Here's a start to creating a supply of healthy basics (whenever possible, make it organic). Many of these ingredients are used in the recipes offered in this chapter:

- Canned black beans and chickpeas
- Dried lentils
- Quinoa
- Coconut oil and olive oil
- Nuts and seeds, including almonds, walnuts, cashews, sunflowers, pumpkin seeds, chia seeds, hemp seeds, and flax seeds
- Tofu
- Hearty fresh greens like kale and spinach
- Soy, almond, or cashew milk
- Nut butters

Breakfast

Bodacious Berries

Skipping breakfast is a big no-no. If your tummy isn't smitten with the idea of a heavy, protein-rich breakfast, opt for a smoothie.

Makes 5 cups

1 cup cranberry or pomegranate juice

1 cup nondairy milk such as silken tofu, soy, almond, or coconut milk

2 cups organic frozen berries (such as blueberries, raspberries, and blackberries, alone or in any combination)

2 tablespoons real maple syrup (optional)

Mix all ingredients in the blender for a full minute at high speed until smooth and creamy. Enjoy immediately (recommended) or store in fridge for up to 24 hours.

Jolly Greenie

Makes 5 cups

1 cup organic green grapes

1 large organic green apple, unpeeled and cut in chunks

1 cup organic honeydew melon, cut in chunks

1 cup organic, 100-percent-natural apple cider

Mix all ingredients in the blender for a full minute at high speed until smooth and frothy. Enjoy immediately (recommended) or store in fridge for up to 24 hours.

Date with Almonds Dream

This smoothie also makes a perfect late-afternoon snack, if you need an energy boost.

Makes 5 cups

½ cup whole organic almonds

1 cup organic pitted dates, packed

⅓ cup dark chocolate cocoa powder

1 cup boiling water

1 cup nondairy milk such as silken tofu, soy, almond, or coconut milk

10 ice cubes

Put the almonds, dates, cocoa, and water in the blender. Cover and let the mixture rest, unblended, for 5 to 10 minutes. Add the nondairy milk and ice cubes and blend for a full minute at high speed until the smoothie is thick and yummy. Enjoy immediately (recommended) or store in fridge for up to 24 hours.

- -

Treat Yourself to Chocolate

Research on the indigenous Kuna Indian population of Panama suggests that unprocessed cocoa may be the healthiest form, due to its high flavonol content. Since flavonols are destroyed through chemical Dutch-processing, or alkalization, look for cocoas labeled "natural," as they have not been treated with alkali.

- -

Tasty Tropics

Makes 5 cups

1 cup organic coconut milk

5 cups cubed organic mango, papaya, pineapple, and/or peaches

1 organic frozen banana (sliced in thirds)

Mix all of the ingredients in the blender for a full minute at high speed until smooth. Enjoy immediately (recommended) or store in fridge for up to 24 hours.

Magnificent Muesli

Makes 4 cups

1 cup plus 2 tablespoons rolled oats

2 tablespoons oat bran

¼ cup organic raisins

3 tablespoons chopped organic walnuts

1 tablespoon raw organic sunflower seeds

real maple syrup, to taste

In a large bowl, combine the oats, bran, raisins, walnuts, and seeds. Drizzle in the maple syrup. Mix well.

Quinoa Pudding

Makes 2 cups

1 cup quinoa

2 cups water

2 cups organic apple juice

1 cup organic raisins

2 tablespoons lemon juice

1 teaspoon ground cinnamon

salt, to taste

2 teaspoons vanilla extract

Place the quinoa in a sieve and rinse thoroughly. Allow it to drain, then place the quinoa in a medium saucepan with the water. Bring to a boil over high heat. Cover the pan, lower the heat, and simmer until all the liquid is absorbed and the quinoa is soft (approximately 15 minutes). Add the apple juice, raisins, lemon juice, cinna-

mon, and salt. Cover the pan and simmer for another 15
minutes. Stir in the vanilla extract. Serve warm.

• •

The United Nations General Assembly declared 2013 as
the International Year of Quinoa.

• •

Yummy Pancakes

2 servings (4 pancakes)

1 cup rye flour

1 tablespoon soy flour

1 ½ teaspoons baking powder

⅛ teaspoon salt

⅛ teaspoon ground cinnamon

½ teaspoon vanilla extract

½ cup soy milk

½ cup water

¼ cup chopped organic pecans

½ tablespoon olive oil

1 pat butter

real maple syrup, to taste

In a medium bowl, stir together the rye flour, soy flour,
baking powder, salt, and cinnamon. Make an indentation
in the middle of the flour mixture and pour in the vanilla,
soy milk, and water. Mix until all of the dry ingredients
have been absorbed. Stir the pecans into the batter. Heat
a large skillet over medium heat and coat it with olive oil
and butter. Add more of either if necessary to keep the

skillet greased. Pour about ⅓ cup of batter onto the hot surface, and spread out to approximately a ¼-inch thickness. Cook until bubbles appear on the surface, then flip and brown on the other side. Drizzle with maple syrup to taste. Serve warm.

Fruity Salad

4 servings

6 pineapple chunks, with juice

1 medium organic red apple, peeled, cored, and diced

1 medium organic orange, peeled and diced

1 medium banana, sliced

⅓ cup seedless organic grapes, halved

Toss the pineapple chunks, apple, orange, banana, and grapes together in a large bowl and serve.

•••

Easy Mid-Morning or Late-Afternoon Snack Suggestions

- Sliced apples and cinnamon
- Roasted chickpeas
- Trail mix. Choose your organic dried fruits, nuts, and seeds, and add some organic dark chocolate chips and goji berries. Place it all in an airtight glass or plastic container and shake.
- Bowl of berries with a dollop of cashew butter
- Celery with almond butter and goji berries
- Dates stuffed with cashew or peanut butter

•••

Mid-Morning Pick-Me-Ups

Beet Smoothie

Serves 1

1 (15-ounce) can beets, including juice

1 cup silken tofu

Mix all ingredients in the blender for a full minute at high speed until smooth and sweet.

•••

The beetroot comes in many colors: Red, golden, and chi-oggia beets are grown for eating, white beets are mostly grown for producing beet sugar, and yellow beets are grown for livestock feed.

•••

Lunch

It's a good idea to consider lunch your main meal as opposed to dinner. This way you won't digest while you sleep. Here are some suggestions:

Fast Vegetable Curry

Serves 2

1 medium yellow onion, halved and thinly sliced

1 teaspoon olive oil

2 garlic cloves, crushed

1 tablespoon grated fresh ginger

1–3 cups chopped fresh firmer vegetables of your choice (such as potatoes, cauliflower, or broccoli)

2–3 teaspoons curry paste

salt, to taste

1 (14-ounce) can organic coconut milk

generous handful of fresh spinach, chopped

In a large skillet set over medium-high heat, sauté the onion in the olive oil for 2–3 minutes, until soft. Add the garlic and ginger and cook for another minute. Add a generous handful of any firm vegetable for a few minutes until they soften and start to turn golden on the edges. Add the rest of the veggies with the curry paste, salt, and coconut milk and bring the mixture to a simmer. The length of cooking will depend on the vegetables. When the vegetables are ready, stir in the spinach and cook for a minute, just until it wilts. Serve while hot and yummy!

Vegetarian Chili

Serves 4

1 tablespoon olive oil

2 cups chopped yellow onion

3 garlic cloves, minced

4 cups water, divided

2 tablespoons sugar

2 tablespoons chili powder

2 (14½-ounce) cans diced tomatoes, undrained

1 (15½-ounce) can chickpeas (garbanzo beans), rinsed and drained

1 (15-ounce) can black beans, rinsed and drained

1 (15-ounce) can kidney beans, rinsed and drained

1 (6-ounce) can tomato paste

Heat the olive oil in a large Dutch oven over medium-high heat. Add the onion and garlic; sauté for 3 minutes or until tender. Add 3 cups of the water and the next 6 ingredients, stirring to combine. Combine the remaining cup of water and tomato paste in a bowl, stirring with a whisk until blended. Stir the tomato paste mixture into the bean mixture. Bring to a boil; reduce heat and simmer for 5 minutes or until thoroughly heated.

• •

National Chili Day Is February 27!

• •

Falafel and Avocado

Serves 2

1 (15-ounce) can pinto beans, rinsed and drained

¼ cup (about ¾-ounce) finely crushed whole-grain baked tortilla chips

2 tablespoons finely chopped green onions

1 tablespoon finely chopped cilantro

⅛ teaspoon ground cumin

1 large egg white

1 ½ teaspoons olive oil

Spread:
   ¼ cup mashed peeled avocado

   2 tablespoons finely chopped tomato

   1 tablespoon finely chopped red onion

   1 teaspoon fresh lime juice

   ⅛ teaspoon salt

Remaining ingredients:
   2 (6-inch) whole-grain pitas

   red onion, thinly sliced, to garnish

   handful organic mixed greens

Place the pinto beans in a medium bowl; partially mash them with a fork. Add the next 5 ingredients and stir until they are well combined. Shape the bean mixture into 4 (½-inch-thick) oval patties. Heat the olive oil in a big skillet over medium-high heat. Add the patties to the skillet; cook for 3 minutes on each side or until the patties are browned and thoroughly heated. To prepare spread, combine all the ingredients, stirring well. Place 1 patty in each pita half. Spread about 2 tablespoons of the avocado spread over the patty in each pita half; top with onions and greens.

Marvelous Mango and Shrimp Sensation

Serves 3

   3 tablespoons fresh lime juice

   2 tablespoons olive oil

   2 large ripe but firm mangoes peeled and cut into cubes

2 medium ripe but firm avocados peeled and cut into cubes

⅔ cup thinly sliced green onions

⅔ cup chopped cilantro

1 tablespoon minced fresh hot red or green chile (or ½ teaspoon dried red chile flakes)

1 pound (70 to 110) peeled cooked shrimp

Pour the lime juice into a large bowl and whisk in the olive oil. Add the mangoes and avocados to the bowl. Add the green onions, cilantro, chile, and shrimp. Mix gently. Serve or cover and chill for up to 1 hour.

••

Just Checking: Are You Drinking Enough Water?

A good rule is to drink six to eight 8-ounce glasses of water or other fluid every day.

How can you tell if you're drinking enough water? The simplest way to know if you're getting enough fluid is to check the color of your urine. If it's clear or pale, you're most likely getting enough to drink. However, if it's darker yellow, then you probably need to drink more. Have another glass of water!

••

Lovely Light Dinners

Try to finish your last meal by 7 p.m. so the major work of digestion can be done by the time you tuck into bed. Here are some recipe suggestions.

Roasted Sweet Tater Soup

Serves 2

1 large sweet potato

1 tablespoon olive oil

1 medium yellow onion, chopped

3 garlic cloves, chopped

1 tablespoon finely grated fresh ginger

½ teaspoon curry powder

½ teaspoon ground turmeric

½ teaspoon ground sage

⅛ teaspoon cayenne pepper

1 ½ cups coconut milk

½ quart organic vegetable broth

salt, to taste

Preheat the oven to 400°F. Poke holes in the sweet potato, wrap it in foil, and roast it in the oven for 60 minutes or until very soft. When the sweet potato is finished roasting, allow it to cool then carefully place it in a blender (with skin on). In a medium skillet, heat the olive oil over medium heat and sauté the onion until translucent, about 10 minutes. Add the garlic, ginger, curry powder, turmeric, sage, and cayenne pepper and sauté for another 2 minutes. Add this mixture to the blender with the sweet potato, along with the vegetable broth and coconut milk. Blend until smooth. Add the soup back into the sauté pan (or large pot) to heat it to desired temperature. Add salt, to taste.

Ordering in a Restaurant

There's no reason why you can't enjoy meals in restaurants while sticking to a healthy meal plan. Here are tips to help you stay on track:

- As a beverage choice, ask for water.
- Start your meal with a salad packed with veggies, to help control hunger and feel satisfied sooner.
- Ask for simple olive oil and vinegar as a salad dressing—and on the side.
- Choose main dishes that include vegetables, such as stir-fries.

If main portions at a restaurant are larger than you'd like, try one of these strategies to keep from overeating:

- Order an appetizer or a side dish instead of an entrée.
- Share a main dish with a friend.
- If you can chill the extra food right away, take leftovers home in a "doggy bag."
- Resign from the "clean your plate club." When you've eaten enough, leave the rest.
- Order fruit for dessert.

Savory Salmon Salad

This recipe works great when you're in a super hurry!

Serves 2

1 (7½-ounce) can wild salmon, drained, skin and large bones removed

1 tablespoon olive oil

1 small garlic clove, minced

2 drained oil-packed sun-dried tomatoes, finely chopped

5 pitted kalamata olives, finely chopped

2 green onions, finely chopped

1 teaspoon balsamic vinegar

water, as needed

salt and freshly ground black pepper, to taste

1 ripe but firm avocado, pitted and halved

1 tablespoon pine nuts

In a bowl, combine the salmon, olive oil, garlic, sun-dried tomatoes, olives, green onions, and vinegar; mash with a fork. Add a little water to adjust the texture, if necessary. Season with salt and pepper. Spoon salmon salad into avocado halves. Sprinkle with pine nuts.

Peachy Arugula Salad

Serves 4

4 cups arugula

2 medium peaches, pitted and sliced into thin wedges

1 medium green bell pepper, finely chopped

⅓ cup slivered almonds

1 tablespoon olive oil

1 tablespoon balsamic vinegar

½ tablespoon fresh-squeezed orange juice

salt, to taste

cayenne pepper, to taste

To make the salad, combine the arugula, peaches, bell pepper, and almonds in a large bowl. Whisk together the oil, vinegar, orange juice, salt, and cayenne pepper in a separate bowl for your dressing. Just before serving, the toss salad with the dressing.

Time to Tuck In

Ahhh…ready to tuck in but still feeling edgy? Here are some teas that will help you relax and catch those crucial zzz's.

Best Bedtime Teas

Catnip. The big reason catnip tea is a good tea to drink before bedtime is that it acts as a natural muscle relaxer and stress reducer. Catnip enhances sleep because it alleviates or lessens conditions that disrupt sleep, like headaches, cramps, and indigestion. Caution: Don't sip catnip if you're pregnant.

Chamomile. This tea is known to calm nerves and is a safe alternative to other sleep aids, even for children.

Jasmine. This tea relieves headaches and calms the body, helping you to wind down before bedtime.

Peppermint. Peppermint teas have a number of medicinal qualities to help conditions that can interfere with restful sleep, such as a nervous stomach, nausea, and other digestive and intestinal problems. A cup of peppermint tea at night naturally de-stresses the body, preparing it for a restful night's sleep.

Sage. Drinking sage tea before bedtime relaxes the stomach and the mind, preparing the body to enjoy a good night's sleep.

nine

and beyond...

It is not in the stars to hold our destiny but in ourselves.

—WILLIAM SHAKESPEARE

Will this be the year you stay on a healthy diet, give stress the boot, get enough sleep, pamper yourself with feel-good treatments, embrace meditation, spend time with friends, open your heart to love, count your blessings, accept change with ease, and ultimately remain steadfast in your desire to live the best life you possibly can?

Well, dear friend, although I hope you do, you're the one steering your life. To help you along, this chapter points you in the direction of techniques that encourage optimum wellness for your body, mind, and spirit.

Body

You probably don't need to be reminded that your body is the temple housing your spirit. If you've gotten through the cleanse you know this is a fact; you've personally experienced it. Now is the ideal time to introduce methods to support your body's present well-being. Try them out. If any particular one resonates strongly within, make it part of your regular routine or use it whenever your body tells you it's time.

Progressive Muscle Relaxation

Progressive muscle relaxation (PMR) is a terrific technique to help you reduce tension all over your body, from the top of your head to the bottom of your feet. Follow these PMR steps:

1. Choose a place where you know you won't be interrupted and can relax in peace. Lie down on your back and stretch out somewhere comfortable, whether it's your bed, couch, carpeted floor, or yoga mat.

2. Progressive muscle relaxation focuses sequentially on the major muscle groups. Tighten each muscle and maintain the contraction for 20 seconds before slowly releasing it. As the muscle relaxes, concentrate on the release of tension and the sensation of relaxation. Start with your facial muscles and then work down the body in the following order:

- *Forehead.* Wrinkle your forehead and arch your eyebrows. Hold; then relax.
- *Eyes.* Close your eyes tightly. Hold; then relax.
- *Nose.* Wrinkle your nose and flare your nostrils. Hold; then relax.
- *Tongue.* Push your tongue firmly against the roof of your mouth. Hold; then relax.

- *Face.* Squeeze your features into a grimace. Hold; then relax.
- *Jaw.* Clench your jaw tightly. Hold; then relax.
- *Neck.* Tense your neck by pulling your chin down to your chest. Hold; then relax.
- *Back.* Arch your back. Hold; then relax.
- *Chest.* Breathe in as deeply as you can. Hold; then relax.
- *Stomach.* Tense your stomach muscles. Hold; then relax.
- *Buttocks and thighs.* Tense your buttocks and thigh muscles. Hold; then relax.
- *Arms.* Tense your biceps. Hold; then relax.
- *Forearms and hands.* Tense your arms and clench your fists. Hold; then relax.
- *Calves.* While standing, press your feet down. Hold; then relax.
- *Ankles and feet.* Pull your toes up. Hold; then relax.

The entire routine should take 12 to 15 minutes. If you practice it twice daily, you can expect to master PMR and experience full relief of bodily stress in about two weeks.

• •

Give Your Jaw Special TLC

A lot of us carry major tension in our jaw, often unknowingly. To loosen the tension, open your mouth wide for half a minute or so, breathing naturally through your nose. When you feel you've released the tension, allow your mouth to gently close.

• •

Legs Up-the-Wall (Viparita Karani) Yoga Pose

Just as important as strenuous yoga poses are restorative positions. The following pose is a perfect antidote to an overworked body. For support you'll need one or two thickly folded blankets or a firm round bolster. If you're naturally more flexible, use a higher support that is closer to the wall. Your distance from the wall also depends on your height: if you're shorter move closer to the wall; if you're taller move farther from the wall. Experiment with the position of your support until you find the placement that works for you and creates a comfy position.

1. Sit sideways on the right end of the support, with your right side against the wall. Exhale, and with one smooth movement, swing your legs up onto the wall and your shoulders and head lightly down onto the floor. The first few times you do this you may slide off the support and plop down with your buttocks onto the floor. Don't get discouraged. Try lowering the support and/or moving it slightly farther off the wall until you master the movement, then move back closer to the wall.

2. Next, raise and release the base of your skull away from the back of your neck and soften your throat. Don't push your chin against your sternum; instead let your sternum lift toward the chin. Take a small roll (made from a towel, for example) and place it under your neck if the cervical spine feels flat. Open your

shoulder blades away from the spine and release your hands and arms out to your sides, palms up.

3. Try to keep your legs pretty firm so they'll stay vertically in place, but don't allow any part of your body to tense up. Release the heads of the thigh bones and the weight of your belly deeply into your torso, toward the back of the pelvis. Soften your eyes and turn them down to look into your heart.

4. You can remain in this pose for up to 15 minutes, but try not to release before five minutes are up. When you're ready, be sure not to twist off the support when coming out. Instead, slide off the support onto the floor before turning to the side. You can also bend your knees and push your feet against the wall to lift your pelvis off the support. Then slide the support to one side, lower your pelvis to the floor, and turn to the side. Stay on your side for a few breaths, and come up to a sitting position with an exhalation.

Breathe Deeply

One of the simplest ways to relieve tension is with deep breathing. Here's an easy exercise to put deep breathing into practice:

1. Lie on your back with a pillow under your head. Bend your knees (or put a pillow under them) to relax your stomach.

2. Put one hand on your stomach, just below your rib cage.

3. Slowly breathe in through your nose. Your stomach should feel like it's rising.

4. Exhale slowly through your mouth, emptying your lungs completely and letting your stomach fall.

5. Repeat several times until you feel calm and relaxed.

Listen to Music

Most of us have experienced music's profound effect on our emotions. But in addition to evoking an emotional reaction, music also soothes and relaxes our bodies. Specifically, slow tempos can relax muscles and help release stress. So what type of music works best to reduce muscle tension and stress? For starters, Native American, Celtic, Indian stringed instruments, drums, and flutes are very effective at relaxing the mind and body, even when played moderately loud. Rain, thunder, and nature sounds may also be relaxing, particularly when mixed with other music, such as light jazz, classical (the slow "largo" movement), and easy-listening music. How do you choose the relaxation music that's most effective for you? The answer rests with you: first enjoy the music being played, and then discover firsthand whether it relaxes you. Forcing yourself to listen to relaxation music that irritates will only create tension, not reduce it.

Take a Bath

Lots of us prefer to take a shower rather than "waste" precious time soaking in a tub. Sound familiar? But you might be persuaded to take a warm, relaxing bath at least once a week after you learn about its surprising health benefits. Not only does bathing relieve stress and tension, it can also detoxify, stimulate circulation, and boost your immune system. Plus, a warm bath helps muscles to relax as well as helps to increase their elasticity, especially when followed with gentle stretching. The benefits of bathing to the musculoskeletal system may even reduce trips to the chiropractor by helping to maintain muscle position and equalizing tension on the skeletal system. In addition, a good soak can relieve tension headaches.

A long soak in a tub can also help anxiety and allow worries to float away. A study conducted in Osaka, Japan, confirmed the stress-relieving effects of bathing. Two sensitive salivary stress markers, cortisol and chromogranin, were measured before and after subjects bathed for 60 minutes. The researchers found a marked reduction in these stress markers. You can bathe for less than 60 minutes, but plan to soak in your bath without interruption.

Make your bath warm enough to induce a sweat but not hot enough to scald you. The process of perspiration removes toxins from the body. You may even notice that a regular bath routine reduces perspiration odor so you have less need for deodorants. The heat of the water also kills many strains of bacteria and viruses, decreasing the number of colds and infections you may get throughout the year.

Bonus: Bathing increases blood circulation by increasing the rate of nourishing blood cells to damaged tissue. In addition, dead cells are removed from the body more quickly, increasing the ability to stay healthy and energetic. Bathing can also help fight infection and colds. The vascular and lymph system stimulation decreases your risk of colds and infection by stimulating the immune system, thus improving your body's ability to destroy the bacteria and virus cells that can make you sick.

••

Caution: If you have high or low blood pressure, a bath that is too hot may cause problems. Also, allow the water to cool or add cold water slowly to return your body temperature and circulation to normal before getting out of a hot bath.

••

Try Aromatherapy

A growing body of evidence points to the positive effect of aromatic essential oils in treating a wide variety of conditions from easing tensions and healing wounds to revitalizing the skin and spirit. Here's a round-up of the most popular scents:

Tea tree oil. This oil is reported to make white blood cells more active, thereby boosting the immune system. It's widely recognized as a powerful tool against a variety of harmful bacteria, viruses, fungi, molds, and parasites.

Lavender. Studies published in the likes of *Human Psychopharmacology* show inhaling lavender oil is more effective for insomnia than a placebo. For best results, use topically or add 10 drops to bathwater. Sheets washed in water containing lavender oil may also promote sleep. Although nontoxic, the scent may trigger nausea if too much is used.

Eucalyptus. This herb's aroma is the key ingredient in Vicks VapoRub and, not surprisingly, is a treatment for respiratory complaints. Need we say more?

Peppermint. This oil has been shown to relieve pain when applied externally to sore muscles. It may also fight fever and help to ease headaches and respiratory infections. Use only a small amount of oil topically or in bathwater. Caution: Keep eyes closed when inhaling its scent and wash hands thoroughly after use, as the oil can also be an irritant.

Chamomile. Mostly known for its calming effects as a tea, it's also believed to reduce inflammation and fight skin infections. Use topically or add six to 10 drops to running bathwater.

Ginger. Noted for its warming and decongestant properties, ginger also helps fight off colds and flu and reduces fever by inducing perspiration. For best results, mix the powder with olive oil and massage into the chest and inhale. Or you can add six drops of the ginger powder and olive oil to running bathwater. Make sure to dilute it to avoid skin irritation.

Mind

We live in the era of distraction. There's Facebook, Instagram, Twitter, emails, texts, and Skype, not to mention binge television programming, 24-hour news, and advertising on just about every surface. All this information means we're either looking at the past or projecting into the future and feeding our desires. That's a big problem because the secret to joy is to be fully in the present. Living in the here and now isn't easy, but it's worth trying to attain. It reduces the kinds of impulsivity and reactivity that underlie depression, binge eating, anxiety, and attention deficit problems.

The following everyday activities, if done with mindfulness, can change your life.

Mindful Walking

Walking meditation can be practiced in different ways, requiring varying levels of concentration. While walking at a normal pace may be just right for developing concentration, very slow walking is more effective for achieving deeper awareness. So, you may want to experiment with walking at slightly different paces until you find one that feels right for you. As with any meditation method, skill in walking meditation comes from practice and patience. Here's a good introduction:

- Choose a path with a clear beginning and end. The walking path can be either inside or outside, depending upon your preference and the area available. That said, quiet surroundings in nature are best.
- Whenever possible, it is better to practice in bare feet, although this is not essential.
- Pick an appropriate time and decide how long to walk mindfully. Between 15 and 20 minutes is enough for a beginner.
- Stand at one end of the path and hold your hands gently together in front of your body. Your eyes remain open, gazing down along the path about two yards ahead. The intention is not to be looking

at anything in particular but simply to see that you remain on the path and know when to turn around.

- Try to put aside all concerns for the past and future. In order to calm the mind and establish awareness in the present, abandon any preoccupation with work, home, and relationships, and bring the attention to your body.

- Walk at a slow, relaxed pace, being fully aware of each step until you reach the end of the path you are walking on. Begin with the right foot. While taking that step, pay careful attention to the movement of your foot as it is raised off the ground, moved through the air, and placed on the ground again. Then take a step with your left foot, being equally attentive. Continue walking in this mindful and methodical way until you have reached the end of the path.

- If, while walking, you become aware that your mind has wandered away from the step, say internally, "Okay, distraction," and gently, but firmly, bring your attention back to the step. It is often helpful to make a mental note of "right" and "left" with each corresponding step, as this keeps the mind more involved with the act of walking.

- When you arrive at the end of your path, stop for a moment and check to see what the mind is doing. Is it being attentive? If necessary, reestablish awareness.

- Now turn and walk back to the other end in a similar fashion, remaining mindful and alert. Continue to pace up and down for the duration of the meditation period, gently making an effort to sustain awareness and focus attention on the process of walking.

Mindful Cleaning

Lots of us complain when we're faced with household chores, particularly cleaning. But setting your mind on cleaning without judgment is a way to bring what you once wanted to avoid into an activity you can embrace fully. To make this chore mindful, begin with these overall principles:

- **Just clean.** Don't think about what you have to do next. And don't opt for distractions such as listening to the radio or keeping the TV on in the background. Just do what you're doing—dusting, vacuuming, washing the floors. Just do it.

- **Be grateful.** This is an excellent time to be grateful for what you have, for having the ability to clean or declutter. You can be grateful for all the material possessions in your home and of course, more importantly, the people in your life. If they share your home, offer them the gift of making their life easier by taking care of these chores and creating a spiffy environment.

- **Pay attention.** Practice focusing on the sound of the vacuum, the swipe of the broom against the floor, the dust being wiped clean from the surface. Notice when your mind is wandering. Bring it back. Notice how your body is moving, the way you're breathing. Experience whatever is happening in this moment and wipe it clean.

Mindful Eating

Mindful eating was briefly mentioned when discussing how to return to food consumption after the MC. But now that you're back in the swing of eating three square meals a day, you have an even greater opportunity to make your meals an exploration of mindfulness. Here's how to do it:

- **Start small.** Wild expectations usually lead to defeat. Like all new habits, it's best to set small goals at first. Choose one meal or snack each day when you can commit to focusing on mindful eating.

- **Stop multitasking at mealtimes.** It's really difficult to focus on eating if you're doing other things. Set aside time for eating without other entertainment.

- **Only eat at the table.** Another way to minimize mindless munching is to get into the habit of eating only when you are sitting down and able to give the food your full attention. No more snacking on the run.

- **Appreciate appearances.** There's beauty in the food right in front of you. Take a moment to really look at what you're about to eat. Taking the time to notice sets the scene for mindful eating.

- **Focus on each mouthful.** Think about the flavor, texture, and even the sound of the food in your mouth. Focus on how much you like or dislike these sensations.

- **Chew.** While it can be overkill to go to the monastic extreme of 100 bites per mouthful, make sure you chew your food enough so that it is well broken down before you swallow.

- **Use cutlery and put it down between mouthfuls.** It's much easier to make each bite mindful when using a knife and fork. Of course if you feel like you're having a ridiculous *Seinfeld* moment eating a dark chocolate bar with utensils, then skip this step, but do put the bar down in between bites so you can still focus.
- **Talk and share.** One of the joys of eating is sharing a meal with loved ones. It can be challenging to incorporate mindfulness in a social situation but not impossible. Turn the focus of the conversation to the meal while you are actually eating. Share what you are experiencing in terms of flavors and textures, likes and dislikes.
- **Opt for quality not quantity.** By choosing smaller amounts of the best food you can afford, you will not only enjoy it more, you're far more likely to be satisfied without having to overeat.
- **Prepare your own meals, preferably from fresh ingredients.** The cooking process can be as relaxing and enjoyable as eating if you let it. Knowing exactly what has gone into your meal is another expression of mindfulness.

Mindful Listening

We talk a lot, but is anyone really paying attention, tuning in mindfully and truly listening? According to the International Listening Association, an organization that promotes the study and development of listening skills, when it comes to conversation, most of us only take in about half of what's being said. Even though it's tough to stay focused and pay attention, proven techniques can help you be mindful and truly listen. Here are some of them:

- **Avoid giving advice.** It's natural to want to help the speaker by offering a solution or sharing our perspective on a problem. But no matter how carefully we may have weighed our response, experts say once advice is offered, communication is likely to shut down. Instead offer open-ended statements such as, "Take me through the steps that led you here." By staying neutral you not only let the speaker know you're listening but allow her to reach a conclusion she can own.

- **Clear your head.** When someone starts to talk to you, do your best to clear your mind of any thoughts that are occupying you. Remove any sense of judgment about the person who is talking.

- **Don't second-guess.** How many times have you thought or said, "I know what you're thinking"? Resist the urge. If you tune into your intuition, you won't be listening to the speaker. To help you stay in the moment, imagine a total stranger is speaking to you.

- **Fill in the blanks.** Most of us tell only 75 percent of our story. You can perfect your listening skills by tuning into gaps and inconsistencies, but without judgment. Take the perspective of someone who is curious and interested by asking follow-up questions whenever something doesn't make sense.

- **Tune into emotion.** Real listening means noting the emotional content underneath the words. Pay attention to voice inflection, facial gestures, and body language. If you're not sure about underlying emotions you can simply ask, "What are you feeling?"

- **Make eye contact.** There's truth behind the saying "Eyes are the windows to the soul." Recent research into bonding shows eye-to-eye contact between mothers and their babies activates the prefrontal cortex—the area of the brain responsible for attachment. When you make eye contact the lines of communication are deepened; the speaker literally feels heard.

- **Don't think of an answer.** It's impossible to be listening while figuring out how to respond at the same time. If you want to get information from anyone, don't rehearse your answer while they're speaking; keep your attention focused on their words. And when you do respond, avoid parroting or simply repeating sentences word for word. Contrary to popular belief, parroting sends the message you're not truly listening—only hearing.

- **Be patient with silence.** A vacuum gets filled. Even if someone has stopped speaking, allow their words to soak in before responding. Waiting a minute, or even longer, not only allows the listener to really consider what's been said, but gives the speaker a chance to clarify or change thoughts. To show you're still paying attention, lean in and cup your hand under your chin.

- **Fight off distractions.** According to the International Listening Association, research indicates that we spend about 45 percent of our time listening, but we are distracted, preoccupied, or forgetful about 75 percent of that time. One of the most important ways to listen, especially in this age of computers and smartphones, is to simply shut them off and bring your full presence to the situation.

Spirit

Keep a Journal

During the course of your day it's natural for a million thoughts and memories to swirl around. You may envision a new project, remember an event from your childhood, appreciate a sunset, or feel sudden tenderness toward an old friend. Writing down your thoughts and keeping a journal is a way to practice mindfulness by recording and embracing your life. You can use your journal as a private way to explore your thoughts and delve into your psyche, or you may choose to share it with others. Many people write as a way to share their personal history. But the most important part of writing in your journal is that it offers you a chance to be utterly truthful and present. Use it as a safe place to go during quiet times. Know that it is your private possession. There is a reason why many journals are designed with locks and keys. But it doesn't matter whether you buy a nice, bound notebook; the aim is to just let your words flow. Keeping a journal is a personal journey that can help you delve into your consciousness. Here are some ways to get the most out of one.

- **Do it routinely.** It's important to try and write every day or at least once a week. The important thing is that instead of allowing important thoughts pass you by, you pay attention and write them down. Remember, these writings are not for publication (unless you choose them to be) so you need not fret about the sentence structure or, more importantly, the subject matter. You will be less inhibited if your writings are just between you and the notebook paper.
- **Explore.** Writing gives you the opportunity to take stock of yourself, think about how you feel, and express your opinions. Think of it as a forum for self-analysis. Try not to dwell on negative emotions. If those are the only ones you explore, try learning something about what you are feeling and imagine ways to let go of your emotional attachment. Write down these thoughts, too.
- **Collect the words of others.** Affirmations, biblical proverbs, poems, excerpts from stories, even song lyrics with special significance can be recorded in your journal.
- **Be expansive.** If you're a visual person, you may decide to draw or cut out images and paste them in your notebook; you can use these for inspiration.

Let Go of a Grudge

Grudges have a way of digging in and sticking like Velcro. They might feel good at first, but the feeling soon sours.

Grudges can not only make you feel emotionally bitter and resentful, but damage your spirit and also affect your physical health. Studies show this kind of seething anger increases heart rate, elevates blood pressure, and makes us flat-out depressed. The good news? There are ways to release a grudge. The first step is simply seeing that you're holding onto a grudge and acknowledging it. From there, take the following steps:

- **Don't forgive until you are really ready.** You don't want to be sweeping your feelings under a rug of hidden resentment.
- **Ask for an apology.** Although an apology won't change what caused your hurt, it can help ease it, and it's certainly okay to ask for one if you think it will help you to heal.
- **Talk to someone.** If you believe someone has done you wrong, discuss it with a trusted friend and get her viewpoint. A different perspective may open an avenue of forgiveness.
- **Write down your thoughts.** Think about what upsets you and how you feel about it. Writing can keep your perspective in focus.
- **Don't focus on righting the wrong—or getting revenge.** Although this is a common reaction of grudge-holders, it's a destructive pattern. Instead, practice releasing your anger through exercise, talk therapy, or deep breathing and meditation.
- **Remind yourself: Letting go of a grudge does not mean you stuff your feelings away.** It means changing how you think about the situation. You can't

change what happened, but you can change your attitude and interpretation of events.

- **Remind yourself that you're not perfect.** How many times have you made a mistake?

Letting go of a grudge doesn't mean you're condoning a hurtful action, or excusing bad behavior; it means you're moving on so that you can put emotional control back in your own hands.

Practice Loving-Kindness

In a culture that prides itself on competition and individuality, sometimes loving-kindness is put on the back burner. But compassion toward oneself and others is a positive tool benefiting our spirits—and more. Open your heart and you'll:

- **Reduce your stress response.** A study from Emory University concluded that compassionate meditation lessened inflammatory responses to stress, which in turn was a means of reducing depression, heart disease, and diabetes.
- **Find making changes is easier.** Unsavory habits—whether they consist of anger, laziness, procrastination, or overeating—tend to stick even harder when we identify them as parts of ourselves that we don't like. But studies show when we turn toward bad habits with loving-kindness and understanding, they're easier to release.
- **Release judgment.** Are you Judge Judy? If you find yourself scrutinizing others harshly, there's a good chance your inner critic is also hard at work.

Developing compassion and loving-kindness releases both your inner and outer critic.

- **Boost your self-esteem.** Studies consistently show that those who rate highest on scales of self-esteem are also the most compassionate. It makes sense. Why does it make sense? Because in order to love and accept others, you need to feel the same way about yourself.

- **Catch more zzz's.** When something eats away at you—whether it's a person or event—it can keep you tossing and turning. Tucking in with a full heart of acceptance and loving-kindness means your mind is calm and you'll be more likely to have a good night's sleep.

Stay Calm

I'm a little uneasy admitting this, but here it goes: I'm not your go-with-the-flow type. In fact, despite my decades-long yoga practice, daily meditation, and detox dieting, I can get floored by a case of the nerves. Everything from being stuck in traffic to tackling a new recipe can unhinge me. Are there ways to chill out? Although nail-biters can't expect to be cured forever, proven techniques can bring temporary calm. Check these out:

- **Leave the drama to Meryl Streep.** In other words, try not to catastrophize. Instead of saying things like, "This is too much. I can't deal with it," try telling yourself, "It's no big deal" and "I can get through it."

- **Keep your nerves to yourself.** Standard wisdom has been to talk about our fears, but sometimes it's better to take time to figure things out for ourselves and strategize. Even talking it over with our best friends can backfire since they may tend to sympathize with our anxieties and inadvertently fuel fear.

- **Use your imagination.** Visualizing ways to bring calm can really help. I try to imagine putting my problem in a box, closing it up, and then giving it wings so it can fly away into the clouds, getting smaller and smaller until it disappears. You can come up with your own imagery.

- **Think about what "he or she" would do.** Do you know someone who you would describe as unflappable? Try to think of what this person would do in your situation.

- **Opt to be distracted.** Instead of ruminating, find something fun, engaging, and constructive to do. Take a break and watch a funny movie or read a blog that always make you laugh. When you lighten up, it's a lot easier to keep your cool.

- **Take some wise words.** Certain quotes can center me almost immediately, such as "In three words I can sum up everything I've learned about life: *It goes on*" (Robert Frost) or "If you don't know where you are going, any road will get you there" (Lewis Carroll). But if these don't resonate within you, find quotes or affirmations that do and repeat them to yourself for a quick, calm fix.

Final Quiz:
Calculate Your Energy Quotient

Now that your MC adventure has come to a close, why not check out your energy level? If it's still a bit sluggish, put some of the techniques offered at the end of your analysis into practice for one month, then retake the quiz to see how much more zest you've gained.

According to Jacob Teitelbaum, MD, author of *From Fatigued to Fantastic*, more than 10 percent of Americans have the feeling of disabling fatigue at any given time, and almost 65 percent of us say we just don't have the energy we need. Everyone has a unique energy quotient: a combination of emotional balance, physical well-being, and healthy relationships. In order to truly be at your optimum energy level, you need to take care of all three essentials in your life. This test will help you to discover what you need to zoom in on what you're lacking and ultimately boost your EQ.

1. **You're spending the weekend in a secluded cabin nestled beside a lake in the forest. You pack:**
   a. Hiking boots and a swimsuit.
   b. A journal and lots of film.
   c. Your cell phone and laptop.

2. **When the alarm rings, you:**
   a. Lie awake making a mental list of activities for the day.
   b. Rise immediately, wondering what the day will bring.
   c. Press the snooze button and pull the covers over your head.

3. For your birthday you'd rather have:
   a. A surprise party thrown in your honor.
   b. Dinner in your favorite restaurant with a loved one.
   c. Amnesia.

4. At the end of a working day, you feel:
   a. A little beat but ultimately satisfied with your accomplishments.
   b. Glad that you can start really living.
   c. Exhausted and desperate to relax.

5. Which of these statements sounds most like you?
   a. When I'm feeling distressed, I talk it over with a friend or loved one.
   b. Often I feel apprehensive or irritable, and I just don't know why.
   c. I refuse to let myself feel down.

6. You drink water:
   a. Whenever you feel thirsty.
   b. To meet the recommended quota of eight 8-ounce glasses per day.
   c. Not often enough.

7. Which of these activities most appeals to you:
   a. Swimming.
   b. Sailing.
   c. Snoozing.

8. Choose the Saturday afternoon closest to your ideal:
   a. Taking a long walk or working out at the gym.
   b. Time with friends or family.
   c. Just hanging out with nothing on your plate.

9. **Do you stay up late when there's something you want to watch on TV, even if you're tired?**
   a. Rarely.
   b. Sometimes.
   c. Frequently.

10. **You mostly crave:**
   a. Protein.
   b. Complex carbohydrates.
   c. Sweet stuff.

11. **When it comes to multivitamins, you take one:**
   a. Daily.
   b. Sometimes—if you're feeling rundown.
   c. Never.

12. **You usually keep your daily schedule:**
   a. Partly booked but with some empty spaces.
   b. Flexible—to change with your mood.
   c. Sacred. Your never break plans.

13. **You feel most rested after how many hours of sleep?**
   a. 6 or less.
   b. Between 6 and 8.
   c. 9 or more.

Scoring

Mostly A's: You have higher energy than most.

A spinning top with sparks of energy flying in every direction, you can keep going without taking a break. You join the approximately 20 percent of the American population who fall into the category of type A personality with a naturally speedy metabolism and upbeat attitude that keeps you surging ahead. Although it's terrific that you've got energy-plus, everyone needs to rebalance once in a while. Here's how to moderate your energy so you can keep going without burning out:

- Get enough shut-eye. Although you might need less sleep than most, try to get to bed at the same time each night and awaken the same time each morning. Research shows everyone (even you!) needs at least seven hours of sleep to function efficiently.
- Take a vitamin B complex supplement. This stress reducing vitamin keeps your energy humming.
- Cut down on caffeine; you don't need it! Limit yourself to one cup a day; try soothing herbal teas instead.

Mostly B's: You're rock steady.

Since moderation is your motto, you try to pace yourself. To others it might appear that your accomplishments are effortless, but that's just because you can tame tough problems without wasting valuable energy. This comes naturally to you because your metabolism, adrenal glands, and body type are all set to release energy moderately and without radical highs or lows. But there are rare occasions when even you get stressed out. Recognize the signs—exhaustion, headaches, backaches, short temper, or sleeplessness. That's when it's time for you to relax and try these proven rejuvenation techniques:

- Acupinch. Apply slight pressure and rub your outer ear with your thumb and first finger. This ancient acupressure point is a prime meridian for relaxing muscle tension from the body.

- Breathe deeply for 60 seconds—and watch your breath. This technique sends oxygen to your brain cells, giving your mood and thinking power a boost!
- Take a catnap. Studies show just a 10-minute afternoon snooze can be as beneficial as an hour's worth of extra sleep.

Mostly C's: Your energy could use a boost.

Soaking in a warm bath or snoozing on the couch is your idea of heaven, and it's a healthy practice to set aside time to relax. But if you have too little get-up-and-go, it's hard to get stuff done and meet your goals, which in turn can trigger the blues. It's a cycle. Low energy leads to sadness; sadness leads to low energy. Other factors? A lag in energy can be caused by diet, lack of fresh air and light, or too little exercise. Whatever the underlying cause may be, here are simple energy-boosting techniques designed to match your natural EQ.

- Salute the sun three times in a row during the morning hours and get the benefits of mood-boosting light and exercise. You can do these simple yoga stretches in front of a window or outside.
- Take a walk. Studies show just 20 minutes a day spent outdoors can speed your metabolism and uplift your mood.
- Feel your feelings. When stressful situations arise, be authentic with your feelings: let go of blame and keep your attention on what feels good.
- Put it in writing. According to a University of California study, subjects who kept a daily gratitude journal rated 75 percent higher on scales measuring happiness and reported feeling revitalized and full of energy.

• • • • • • • • • • • •

A final thought before closing the book on the Master Cleanse is a quote from venerable spiritual teacher Ram Dass, author of *Be Here Now*:

> "When you get frustrated because something isn't the way you thought it would be, examine the way you thought, not just the thing that frustrates you. You'll see that a lot of your emotional suffering is created by your models of how you think the universe should be and your inability to allow it to be as it is."

index

acknowledgments

My thanks go to Stanley Burroughs, creator of the iconic Master Cleanse, whose commitment to detoxing was groundbreaking and legendary. Appreciation abounds for Katherine Furman, acquisitions editor and visionary at Ulysses, as well as to supportive and conscientious editor Lindsay Tamura, and to Kourtney Joy, for her ever-enthusiastic energy and devotion to getting my books "out there." Special appreciation for my friends in DUMBO, Brooklyn, and Brattleboro, Vermont, who are willing to listen while I blab on about the pros and cons of fasts, diets, superfoods, vegan dishes, and digestion. Finally, endless gratitude goes to my son, Gabe, who sees the details, but points out the bigger picture and more importantly, the wider-viewed lessons. His vista helps me see the light even through the darker times.

about the author

Robin Westen received an Emmy Award for the ABC health show *FYI*. She is currently the medical director for Thirdage.com, the largest health site for baby boomers on the Web. She is the author of *The 2-Day Superfood Cleanse*, *The Metabolism-Boost Cleanse*, *Ten Days to Detox*, the *Harvard Medical School Guide Getting Your Child to Eat (Almost) Anything*, as well as *V is for Vagina*, which is coauthored with Alyssa Dweck, MD. She's written feature articles for dozens of national magazines including *Glamour*, *Vegetarian Times*, *Psychology Today*, *SELF*, *Cosmopolitan*, and others. Robin has been practicing yoga, meditation, and cleansing for over 15 years. She divides her time between Brooklyn and Vermont.